DETOXIFY
FOR LIFE

**How Toxins Are Robbing You of Your Health
and What You Can Do About It**

*Malcolm
Thank you for
your support &
lessons
In Health & Healing*

Dr. John Cline MD, BSc
with Patrick Grant

DETOXIFY FOR LIFE

Dr. John Cline is a remarkable physician. I have seen some of his patients before and after they were treated, and I fully expected that any book he would write about his medical practice would be every bit as impressive as the results he achieved with those patients. I was not disappointed. "Detoxify for Life" is an important contribution to our understanding of chronic illness. It should be a textbook in medical schools and should be consulted by healers everywhere. Basically, Dr. Cline argues that a great many illnesses, physical as well as mental, are caused by the bombardment of the body by toxic minerals, toxic chemicals, and foods to which people are allergic. Even more importantly, he tells us what we can do about this disturbing set of problems.

Abram Hoffer Ph.D., RNCP
M.D. Retired, FRCPC

Dr. John Cline M.D. has done a masterful job of integrating the old naturopathic concept of detoxification with recent understandings of how toxins affect us. John Cline has also done a great service by writing this book. How do I know this? In 1999 I learned from a member of his clinic about the toxin he discusses in Chapter 6. With this priceless information I have since managed to cure hundreds of patients that had previously stumped me. It turned out that I also carried a considerable amount of this toxin and in removing it I reversed two problems of 20 years' duration that I had thought were genetic. Every person on the planet has been affected by one or more of the nine major toxins that John Cline so clearly describes. Do yourself a favor and start detoxifying!

Dr. Jonn Matsen N.D.
-Author of Eating Alive, The Secrets to Great Health and Eating Alive II

When it comes to the treatment of serious chronic illness, Western medicine is all too frequently TILT-ing at windmills. However, Dr. Cline, a western trained physician from Nanaimo, British Columbia, has spent the last twenty years researching and practicing in this field. He has now written an easy to read but thorough summary of the TILT concept (toxin induced loss of tolerance). He describes how chronic illnesses can develop when toxins cause an imbalance in our biological systems, and he gives examples of effective treatments, including detoxification.

In the ten years that I have been referring my patients to Dr. Cline (their illnesses have ranged from chronic fatigue to cancer), I have repeatedly seen remarkable improvements in the health outcomes for these patients and in the quality of their lives. This book is a must-read for all health practitioners and lay people who are realizing that our toxic environment is seriously and negatively impacting our lives as well as the lives of our children, and that it is time for us all to TILT back -- especially by taking in fewer toxins.

Dr. Stephen Faulkner MB, ChB (NZ)
Past President Association of Complementary and Integrative
Physicians of BC, Family Physician, Duncan BC

DETOXIFY
FOR LIFE

**How Toxins Are Robbing You of Your Health
and What You Can Do About It**

ISBN: 978-1-934919-07-1

More Heart Than Talent Publishing, Inc.

6507 Pacific Ave #329
Stockton, CA 95207 USA
Toll Free: 800-208-2260
www.MHTPublishing.com

FAX: 209-467-3260

Cover art by FlowMotion Inc.

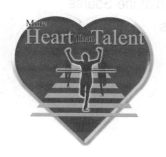

Table of Contents

Foreword

Dr. Cline specializes in the treatment of chronic, complex illnesses. His patients often travel long distances – sometimes, even, from across the world – to visit his clinic in the small town of Nanaimo, on British Columbia's Vancouver Island. They do so because chronic pain has led them to seek the skilled and experienced attention which Dr. Cline can bring to their special kind of suffering.

Our modern world is rapidly becoming ever more toxic as a result of the large scale production of chemicals which have been allowed to contaminate our environment. The toll on human health is likewise becoming increasingly serious, though an individual person's toxic burden can often go un-noticed, because it builds up by small increments over many years. Consequently, when symptoms become manifest they might at first be attributed to more common kinds of disease. A deeper, more adequate investigation requires a careful assessment of how the events of a patient's history, perhaps dating back across decades, might tell the story of a gradually increasing toxic burden. As Dr. Cline's book explains, toxins can continue to build until a tipping point is reached, after which the patient's health tilts into a precipitous decline. The recovery of balance – the equilibrium on which good health depends – requires the kind of patience, courage, and investigative skill which, as this book shows, Dr. Cline brings to the challenging task of helping to restore the health of patients whose suffering has become debilitating.

In partnership with the patient, Dr. Cline therefore works not just to name a disease, but to unearth the genetic and environmental factors that have allowed a specific mischief to harm the patient's health in the first place. Typically, Dr. Cline's investigation focuses on the search for a trigger – often some exposure (such as a toxicant)

– that caused the patient's biological system to crash. Rather than aiming solely to relieve symptoms by way of suppressive medication, Dr. Cline works with the patient to find interventions to restore the underlying balance which has been disturbed

The descriptions of Dr. Cline's search for causes, together with his analyses of particular cases make this book highly engaging, and it is immensely gratifying to learn how the sick can indeed be made whole again. Throughout, in the language of an in-the-trenches clinician, Dr. Cline provides step by step accounts of the process of detoxification and of its indisputable benefits. In short, this is a rich and revealing book, not only for clinicians and for people suffering from chronic pain, but also for general readers who might be interested in the threats to our health caused by the advanced industrial society that in other ways has given us many benefits.

David S. Jones, M.D.

David S. Jones, MD
President, Institute for Functional Medicine
www.functionalmedicine.org

Preface

My name is John Cline, and I am a medical doctor practicing Integrative Medicine on Vancouver Island, British Columbia, Canada. The following book is the culmination of many years of clinical observation, careful listening to what my patients tell me, reading the scientific literature, successfully guiding patients through detoxification programs, and keeping abreast of recent developments by attending a wide variety of courses and conferences.

I first became interested in detoxification many years ago, when my wife and I were faced with a health crisis and seemingly had nowhere to turn. At that time, my wife, Joy, was practically bedridden with fibromyalgia, which is one of the chronic pain disorders. We became increasingly desperate as Joy's health declined despite the treatments provided by our medical system. She tried a number of prescription drugs (from which she often developed side effects); she also tried physiotherapy, acupuncture, chiropractic, massage therapy, dietary changes, counseling, and so on. None of these approaches proved helpful.

My friend and colleague, Dr. Michael Lyon, MD, then suggested that I take training in chelation therapy, which is a safe way to remove toxic metals from the body. Michael's advice turned out to be a revelation for me, and it was the start of my journey into the study of how toxic metals can adversely affect human health. By and by, Joy began getting chelation therapy treatments, and to our surprise and pleasure, her health began to improve. I was then privileged to take a course offered by Dr. Paula Bickle, BSc, PhD on how to safely remove mercury from humans. This course confirmed the value of chelation therapy and set me on the way to a further, committed study of the effects of toxic exposure on human health.

To further assist Joy's recovery, we found a dentist who carefully removed the mercury amalgams (silver fillings) from her teeth. At the same time, she began a heavy metal detoxification program that included the judicious use of DMPS chelation (more about this later). Within a few months of these key interventions, Joy had recovered by approximately 95 percent. I have continued to study in this area and treat patients accordingly. In the process, I learned much of what is recorded in this book.

In May 2000, I attended a conference in Lexington, Kentucky, and while riding in a taxi to the hotel, I was addressed from the back seat by a fellow traveler who spoke with a French-Canadian accent: "Do you know what the TILT Phenomenon is?" I admitted that I had not heard of this concept. The man asking the question was Dr. Jacques Imbeau, DMD, a French-Canadian dentist practicing in New Zealand, and who also had come to Kentucky to participate in the conference. Dr. Imbeau explained that TILT is an acronym for Toxin Induced Loss of Tolerance, meaning that when our bodies accumulate enough toxicants, a tipping point, or tilt, occurs, and our health then deteriorates rapidly in many ways. Until we restore the balance by adequate detoxification, our health will remain impaired.

Subsequently, I came to observe Dr. Imbeau's Tilt Phenomenon in my own patients and found that most of the chronically ill people I interviewed had indeed experienced a gradual increase in toxic load, often over decades; then a seemingly random event would occur – such as a car accident, emotional trauma, metal or chemical exposure or dental work. This event in fact proved to be a tipping point, after which the patient's health suddenly deteriorated, resulting in years of disability. Repeatedly, I have found that identifying the tipping point is crucial for understanding how and why a patient has come to suffer chronically, and in ways that defy conventional diagnoses. When detoxification takes place, it is gratifying to observe how a patient's system tips or tilts back to a healthy equilibrium. I have now observed the Tilt Phenomenon in thousands of patients, and I am forever grateful to Dr. Imbeau for bringing it to my attention.

Each year I am invited to a number of medical conferences to lecture on the subject of detoxification. Throughout my travels, I encounter many people who ask lots of questions, largely because they are desperately searching for answers, either for themselves or for friends and loved ones. I am privileged to be on the teaching faculty of the Institute for Functional Medicine, a group of health practitioners and researchers who are committed to teaching others about a new approach in the assessment and treatment of people suffering with chronic illnesses. Attendance at these conferences is steadily rising, as more health practitioners want to find an effective way to treat the chronic ill health of countless people suffering from exposure to toxic substances. Not surprisingly, an extensive body of literature is developing in the scientific journals, demonstrating what a toxic world we live in and assessing the impact of toxic exposure on humans. Unfortunately, a great deal of this research is given insufficient notice, and its value needs to be better understood.

One woman who attended my clinic is a psychologist. She commented that if I were to work for the rest of my career treating chronically ill people with various forms of detoxification, the number I would be able to treat would be "drops in the bucket" compared to the number actually requiring this kind of approach. She suggested that I write a book so that chronically suffering people could learn that other options are available. I have now taken her advice, which I gratefully acknowledge.

I would like also to thank some others who have enabled this project to come to fruition. I want first to thank my Lord and Savior Jesus Christ who has given me life, a calling, and a purpose, teaching me the joy of serving others while living on this earth. My greatest teacher is my dear wife, Joy, and through her suffering we have both learned a great deal. I thank my daughters Jayme and Jennifer for their love, patience, and support during this project, and I also thank my parents who instilled in me a love of others and a sense of mission.

My professors at the University of Calgary laid the foundational knowledge for all that I do now. Several healthcare practitioners have had a great influence on me including: Dr. Michael Lyon, MD; Dr. Paula Bickle, BSc, PhD; Dr. Dietrich Klinghardt, MD, PhD; Dr. Charles Farr, MD, PhD; Dr. Leonard M. McEwen, MB, PhD; Dr. Anne Sterling Hastings, PhD; Dr. Rashid Buttar, DO, FAAPM, FACAM, FAAIM; Dr. Boyd Haley, PhD; Dr. Peter Brawn, DDS; Dr. Jaques Imbeau, DMD, FACNEM (dental), NZDREX; Dr. Jeff Bland, PhD; Dr. David Jones, MD; and all the staff at the Institute for Functional Medicine. As well, Linda Stone has given wise and timely advice.

I would like also to thank my staff at the Cline Medical Centre for their great dedication and the exceptional care which they offer to the patients who come to us for help. Many thanks also to Erica Combs, President, More Heart Than Talent Publishing, Inc., and Jamie Mattock, Cover & Typesetting Design by FlowMotion Inc. for their hard work, expert guidance, timely advice, and patience in bringing this book to life. Frank Pluta my office administrator performed a lot of the legwork required to move this project along and I am very grateful for his dedicated help. Many thanks as well go to Sharla Clermont who skillfully provided the exquisite illustrations. Lastly, I want to thank the thousands of patients who have attended the Cline Medical Centre over the years for all the lessons they have taught us.

Dr. Patrick Grant, PhD, FRSC, has attended especially to the composition of the text, both by coaching me and by providing the multiple revisions and reworkings which the script required as it evolved towards its final form. Throughout the book I have included a number of cases that I have treated. I have obtained permission from the individuals concerned, and their names have been changed to protect their privacy.

DETOXIFY
FOR LIFE

**How Toxins Are Robbing You of Your Health
and What You Can Do About It**

Introduction - Our Toxic World

Most of us do not realize what a toxic world we live in, or how rapidly our already toxic world is changing for the worse. Each week we hear and read about new sources of toxic exposure and how they can impact our lives. For instance, in 2002 a study was published looking at the levels of toxins found in the stools of newborn babies. The shocking results show significant levels of heavy metals including lead, mercury, and cadmium, as well as a number of insecticides including lindane, malathion, diazinon, parathion, DDT, pentachlorphenol, chlordane, and chlorpyrifos.[1] In 2005, the U.S. Department of Health and Human Services added eleven more compounds to its list of 246 cancer-causing agents in humans,[2] and in all likelihood this already long list will increase as industry continues to produce new chemicals.

A further serious problem arises from the fact that the toxic effects of such chemicals might go largely undetected until extensive damage has been done to people's health, because the symptoms of toxicity often mimic symptoms found in other disease processes. We can therefore carry a significant toxic burden without realizing the harm it is doing to us; meanwhile, we attribute our failing health to other causes. During my many years of medical practice, I have interviewed thousands of people whose illnesses I have been able to trace back to toxic exposures which had previously gone unnoticed. Only when the underlying toxic influences were discovered could treatments be initiated, often producing a remarkable improvement in health.

In describing to patients how toxins affect our health, I often find it useful to refer to the "TILT Phenomenon." As I mention in the Preface, TILT is an acronym that stands for Toxin Induced Loss of Tolerance. It also suggests a tipping point that causes a system to tilt, so that a sudden redistribution of weight occurs. When our cells are exposed to toxic influences, they can resist up to a point, but when they lose their tolerance and begin to fail, a shift or "tilt" occurs. Our intricate cellular processes are then thrown out of balance; consequently, cellular dysfunction and even cellular death can occur, depending on the extent of toxic exposure.

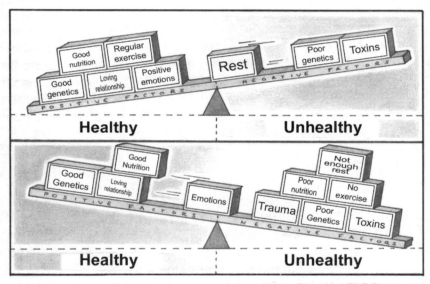

Figure 1.1 TILT Phenomenon

The TILT Phenomenon can be imagined as operating in much the same way as a seesaw or teeter-totter. When two people of equal weight sit on each end of a seesaw, balance is achieved and the seesaw remains horizontal. But if a second person sits on one end, the balance tips and the heavy end hits the ground. If the two people sitting together at the heavy end were then to move closer to the center, the seesaw would gradually regain balance. Most of us have experienced this kind of thing during our playground adventures as children, and I am suggesting that the same process occurs when our cells are exposed to a toxic substance.

For most of us, our toxic burden grows slowly over decades by way of exposure to substances we are used to in our environment, such as herbicides for our lawns, various household cleaning agents, molds in our homes, lead found in multiple products, and even mercury amalgams (silver fillings) in our teeth. When our bodies fail to tolerate the accumulated effect of such ongoing exposure and we reach a tipping point, the resultant imbalance causes a sudden descent into ill health – as if the heavy end of the seesaw were to come crashing onto the ground. Throughout this book I will introduce you to the stories of a number of patients whom I have been privileged to serve, and whose histories illustrate the TILT Phenomenon in operation. In each case, the patient's health declined precipitously after the crucial tipping point was reached, and the challenge was to find a way to restore the balance upon which good health depends.

You will read about:

- Josh, a thirty-six-year-old man with severe muscle pain and fatigue. Josh also had a long history of depression with overlying psychosis which had been treated with strong medications and required multiple hospital admissions.
- Kevin, a fifty-eight-year-old disabled logger who had rheumatoid-like arthritis, Type II diabetes mellitus, angina, and fatigue.
- John, a forty-nine-year-old university professor and consultant with severe chronic fatigue and muscle pain who felt as if he had the flu constantly.
- Daniel, a forty-seven-year-old schoolteacher with a thirteen-year history of chronic fatigue syndrome.
- Heather, a thirty-five-year-old hairstylist who had

suffered with severe hives, muscle pain, and fatigue on a daily basis for twenty-two years.

- Simon, a thirty-nine-year-old aluminum smelter employee who presented with severe eczema and allergies.
- Tom, a sixty-year-old businessman with a long history of fatigue, arthritis, and a recent diagnosis of diabetes mellitus.
- Lori, a forty-three-year-old businesswoman with severe pain and fatigue, who had attempted suicide.
- Richard, a sixty-two-year-old man suffering with polymyalgia rheumatica (a chronic inflammatory condition of the muscles) and experiencing severe pain despite having taken prednisone (a potent steroid drug) for years.
- Dorothy, a fifty-two-year-old nurse who was suffering from fatigue and significant memory disturbances.
- John, a fifty-eight-year-old retired heavy-equipment operator with stiff and sore lower legs and numbness in his feet.

These cases will enable you not only to see how the TILT Phenomenon works, but they will help you to understand the toxic effects of specific substances, the most dangerous of which are dealt with individually in separate chapters.

---

[1] Enrique MO, et al. Prevalence of fetal exposure to environmental toxins as determined by meconium analysis. *Neurotoxicology*. 2002 Sep.23(3):329-39.

[2] Priority List of Hazardous Substances, U.S. Department of Health and Human Services, www.atsdr.cdc.gov/cercla/05list.html.

2

Bodies in Balance - Bodies out of Balance

The basic unit in our bodies is the cell, and each of us has approximately 40 trillion of them. Cells make up tissues, which in turn make up organs. An individual cell functions best if an internal balance is maintained so that the thousands of chemical reactions within each cell can proceed as they should. If a balance is not maintained, the chemical reactions slow down or cease, resulting in disease and cell death.

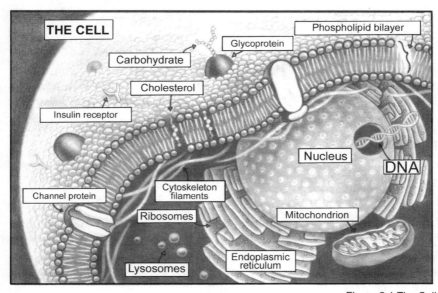

Figure 2.1 The Cell

Unfortunately, because we live in a toxic and stress-filled world, we are bombarded with harmful influences that all too easily disrupt the delicate internal balance necessary for cellular health.

In this chapter I will look briefly at how toxic metals and chemicals, electromagnetic fields, acid/base balance, and the foods we eat can affect the equilibrium that needs to be maintained if we are to thrive. As figure 2.2 illustrates, balance can be affected by positive as well as negative factors. For instance, as we age, unless we are careful about our lifestyle, the balance will tilt invariably into the unhealthy range. The task then is to correct the imbalance by identifying and reducing the negative influences and increasing the positive.

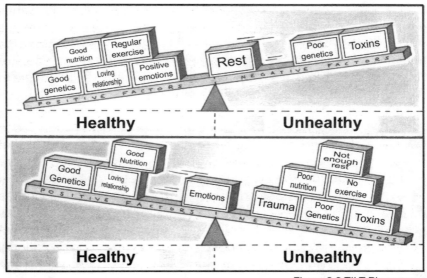

Figure 2.2 TILT Phenomenon

The Cell Membrane

A key factor in promoting healthy cells is the maintenance of the cell membrane, which is the outer covering of the cell, as depicted in Figure 2.1. This membrane protects the cell from unwanted invaders, while also allowing nutrients to enter and waste products to exit. The membrane also serves as an interface between external signals and the inner workings of the cell, and thus acts like a master control mechanism. This membrane also helps to maintain various chemical and electrical gradients and is made up of special types of fats or lipids called phospholipids, which form a double, back-to-back layer called the phospholipid bilayer. The membrane is not rigid, but is constantly moving in a wavelike motion referred to in technical literature as "fluidity." If the membrane loses fluidity, the cell will not function properly.

As we age, and especially if we do not eat well, the structure of the cell membrane tends to become rigid. This, in turn, has a negative effect on the proteins within the cell membrane and consequently on the function of the cell itself. Even more importantly, toxic metals and chemicals have a profound negative impact on cell membrane function and can rapidly tilt the cell membrane into an imbalance. For a basic review of how cells function, more information is available in Appendix A at the end of this book.

Unfortunately, most of us in the industrialized world eat foods that are high in the wrong kinds of fats – that is, fats or oils that have been damaged and altered by processing. These bad fats are usually referred to as hydrogenated fats or trans-fatty acids, and if we avoid them and instead consume good fats, our cell membranes will respond and become healthier. Examples of good oils and fats include omega 3 fish oils, flax oil, virgin olive oil, and virgin coconut oil.[1] Some people also add phospholipids as part of a nutritional supplement program in an attempt to improve cell membrane function.

Phospholipids are especially important for maintaining and improving the function of nerve cells. Because our nervous systems are composed of approximately 60 percent lipids or fats, the regular consumption of the good oils and fats help to improve brain function. (In this sense, we might say that being a "fathead" really is an advantage!) One of the best phospholipids to take orally is phosphatidylcholine, and another is phosphatidylserine.

These introductory remarks can serve to remind us that the cell, which is the basic unit of the body, is highly vulnerable to toxic substances. However, we can improve our body's own detoxification mechanisms by diet and supplementation, and, as we shall see, by a judicious use of chelating agents and far-infrared sauna. Now let me mention briefly some toxic substances that pose a serious threat to the health and balance of our cellular processes.

The U.S. Department of Health and Human Services publishes a Priority List of Hazardous Substances, which indicates that the top three toxicants are arsenic, lead, and mercury.[2] In this book, each of these metals has a chapter devoted to it, but I want now to say something very briefly about mercury, because of its preeminence, and then about some other toxic agents widely dispersed in our environment but often insufficiently noticed. Among these are POPs (Persistent Organic Pollutants), abnormal electrical fields, and the body's acid/base balance.

Mercury

Over 200 symptoms are associated with mercury vapor exposure, and the large majority of these symptoms relate to the nervous system and to impaired energy production. I have treated many people with chronic fatigue, muscle and joint pain, chronic depression and anxiety, memory problems, tremors, hyperactive immune systems manifesting as allergies, asthma, or hives, chronic gastrointestinal disturbances, heart problems, and high blood pressure, as well as many other conditions. By simply getting a load of mercury out of a patient's system, I have repeatedly seen such problems resolve or improve remarkably.

One major difficulty is that chronic low-level exposure to mercury is often so insidious that a person is not aware of the danger. For example, in November 2005, the media reported that in a school in Cranbrook, British Columbia, Canada, many teachers were off work because of mercury poisoning.[3] But how would teachers in a modern high school be exposed to enough mercury to make them sick? The answer lay in a broken barometer in the storeroom of the science lab. The barometer had once been filled with mercury, which leaked after the break occurred. Mercury is one of the few metals that will vaporize at room temperature, and the mercury from the broken barometer behaved accordingly – it turned into vapor and went into the air in the science lab. From there, it was picked up by the ventilation system and spread throughout the school. Eight teachers and many students developed symptoms of mercury toxicity, manifesting with nervous system dysfunction as well as fatigue and muscle pain. When the broken barometer was discovered, mercury levels were tested in the teachers and students, and very high levels were discovered. The school was decontaminated and the affected individuals underwent a series of chelation therapy treatments to pull out the toxic metal. At present, it is too early to tell if there will be permanent consequences for these people as a result of their exposure.

POPs

A second large category of toxicants comprises carbon-based, man-made chemicals that can be stored in the fatty (lipid) tissues in our bodies. Cell membranes, as well as the nervous system (the brain and all the nerves), the hormone secreting glands, and the excretory organs (liver and kidneys), are especially rich in fats and can be especially affected by these toxic chemicals which interfere with important, health-sustaining chemical reactions operating at the cellular level.

In November 2005, a survey was published by the Canadian group, Environmental Defence, in which eleven Canadians from across Canada had their blood tested for eighty-eight different chemicals and metals.[4] The study found evidence that sixty out of a possible eighty-eight toxicants were present in these eleven individuals, with the average being forty-four per test subject. These individuals were all healthy, with no symptoms of environmental toxicity. Yet the toxicants found included heavy metals, DDT, PCBs, stain repellents, and flame-retardants. Older subjects had higher levels of PCBs and pesticides but, strikingly, all tested positive for stain repellents and flame-retardants found in carpets, drapery, and furniture. It is well known that these toxicants are associated with childhood developmental disorders, cancer, hormone disruption, and reproductive and respiratory disorders. As Richard Smith, the executive director of Environmental Defence, says: "If you can walk, talk, and breathe, you are contaminated. Canadians are exposed every day in incredibly insidious ways to harmful toxic chemicals. We are the guinea pigs in a massive, uncontrolled chemical experiment, the disastrous outcome of which is measured in disease and death."[4]

Electrical Balance

If we are to achieve good health, a balance of the body's electrical fields must be maintained. The brain communicates with the rest of the body by sending electrical charges across the cell membranes of nerve cells, and abnormal electrical fields in the body can interfere with this communication. Every cell in our body can be regarded as an organism that needs to eat, drink, breathe, and detoxify itself, and each cell conducts these processes across the cell membrane by taking in nutrients and eliminating waste products. The rate at which substances are exchanged across the membrane determines how efficiently the cell is working. In turn, the rate of exchange depends on the status of the membrane potential, which is the difference in the electrical charge on both sides of the membrane.

The typical cell membrane potential is usually around 80 millivolts (mV), but when the cell has lost its normal membrane potential, the ion pumps and ionic channels in the membrane stop working. In a sense, the cell becomes electrically paralyzed and cannot eliminate its waste products. Abnormal minerals and toxic substances can then accumulate inside the cell, interfering with the ability of the cell to heal itself and restore normal function. If the electrical charge across the membrane is not restored, the cell will often die.

If toxic metals become attached to cell membranes, they will not only negatively impact membrane structure and function but will also adversely affect the electrical charge across the membrane. Other factors that can affect the cell membrane potential include scars on the skin or inside the body, as well as galvanic forces created by the mixtures of metals often found in people's mouths. When scars form, nerve fibers grow into the scars, and because nerves are electrically active, an electric field is created. Sometimes the electric charge produced from scar tissue can be twenty times higher than the usual cell membrane potential (up to 1500 millivolts). This electricity has to go somewhere, and it usually ends up in the nervous system, sending abnormal signals to the brain and thereby causing symptoms to occur that can be quite a distance from the scar itself.

It never ceases to amaze me just how effective scar treatment can be. For example, I treated a woman in her early sixties, who was experiencing a tight sensation in her abdomen and in the muscles around her hips. She was also affected emotionally, and she easily became irritable to a degree that was harming her marriage. When I questioned her, I found that these symptoms began shortly after she had an abdominal hysterectomy. I treated her large, thick, abdominal scar for six weeks with weekly injections of a local anesthetic. Within the first few treatments she noticed a complete resolution of the tight sensation in her abdomen and in her hips. She also told me that she had felt "a cloud lift off me," and her chronic irritability disappeared. She (and her husband) were very much relieved.

In a similar fashion, people frequently experience a sudden improvement when they get their last mercury amalgam removed from their mouths. It is as if an electrical switch has been turned off, as the galvanic forces generated from the metals are suddenly gone. As a further result, people often notice the disappearance of chronic symptoms such as headaches, ringing in the ears, balance problems, and sinus congestion.

There is a growing body of evidence that external electromagnetic fields can also be hazardous to our health because the strength of these fields is often far greater than our bodies were designed to absorb. Exposure to such fields not only has a negative impact on cell membrane potentials, but also on how the nervous system works, and how cells communicate with one another.

Acid/Base (pH) Balance

Another important aspect of keeping the body in balance has to do with the constantly shifting relationship between acids and bases. This relationship is often referred to as pH balance. A simple way to approach this subject is to think of everyday examples of substances that are acidic and substances that are basic, or alkaline. Most of us know that if we were to take a drop of hydrochloric acid and put it on our finger, within seconds a painful sensation would develop as the acid ate through the skin. But if we were to add some baking soda (sodium bicarbonate) to the hydrochloric acid, there would be no problem, because the alkaline baking soda would neutralize the acid.

The same principle applies to the millions of chemical reactions going on in our bodies, producing acidic compounds that, unless neutralized, burn holes in our cell membranes, tissues, and organs. Fortunately, the body has developed sophisticated alkaline substances to neutralize its own acids. However, the typical North American diet consists of many foods that cause the body to produce too many acidic compounds, which in turn have an adverse effect on cell function. Most people who come to my clinic have bodies that are too acidic, a fact that contributes greatly to their chronic health problems. Besides placing these people on diets that are rich in alkaline foods and alkaline minerals, I recommend detoxification to remove heavy metals and organic chemicals. These interventions can have a marked positive effect in shifting the pH balance away from the acidic and towards the alkaline.[5] Certainly, the importance of a balanced diet cannot be overemphasized, and I will digress briefly to illustrate why this is so.

On a recent business trip, I sat next to a woman in her mid-thirties who had great difficulty sitting in the seat because she was adipose challenged (or, in more common language, morbidly obese). She blamed this problem on her "thyroid condition," but it was plain to me from her behavior that much more than a thyroid condition was contributing to her obesity. For instance, she had a handbag filled with M&M's®, cookies, and chips. She then ordered several sodas and informed me that she was addicted to this type of beverage. She also informed me that she stayed away from diet soda because it contained chemicals that are not good for us to consume. She had applied to an insurance company to get funding for stomach bypass surgery but was turned down because she did not fit the criteria. I told her that this was probably a good thing, as there are an increasing number of reports in the scientific literature telling us about the hazards of this type of surgery. In any case, it seemed probable to me that she would not be a good candidate, especially since she seemed to have little interest in changing her eating patterns.

When she found out that I was a physician she asked me for advice, and I informed her about a few simple things to do that I had found worked well with other patients. At the end of my short discourse, and when I had given her some written notes, she pulled out a bag of cookies, explaining that she "had the munchies." She assured me that the cookies were not fattening.

Today, the market is deluged with books on diet, and the topic has become highly confusing. I tell my patients that no one diet will work for everybody, and in the end we have to find what works best for us as individuals. Nevertheless, some important principles do apply to everybody, and a dangerous descent into ill health could well be prevented if my traveling companion – and others like her – would take some basic principles seriously and acknowledge their bad eating habits.

For instance, most patients coming to my clinic do not eat enough protein throughout the day. As you may know, protein is broken down into amino acids, which are the building blocks for most of the structures in our body. Protein is found in all meats, dairy products, chicken, fish, soy, legumes, and many other sources. Instead of consuming adequate amounts of protein, most people eat too many simple sugars, such as those found in refined table sugar, fruits, fruit juices, white rice, bread, potatoes, pasta, and baked goods.

One basic principle of healthy eating is simply to consume adequate amounts of protein and to cut down on sugars and refined carbohydrates, replacing them with the complex sugars found in carbohydrates like vegetables and legumes. Also, it is important to replace bad fats or oils with good fats such as fish oils, extra virgin olive oil, virgin coconut oil, and flax oil. I am frequently struck by the profound improvement in health that people experience when they stop consuming foods that are not good for them.

For instance, one common problem I observe in my patients is dry skin. The skin is a mirror of what is going on inside the body. If the skin is dry, then the trillions of cell membranes will also be "dry," and they won't function as they should. Repeatedly, I have found that dry skin is associated with a deficiency in omega 3 oils. I therefore advise patients to take an adequate dose of fish oil twice a day. Invariably, their skin goes from dry, flaky, and cracked to a smooth, healthy texture because of the simple addition of adequate amounts of fish oil. Yet, all too often I find that people will make changes in their diet only when they are undergoing a health crisis. Otherwise, people's eating patterns are usually difficult to change, not just because of an emotional attachment to foods, but because of years of conditioning that creates bad habits, and also because there is a lack of adequate education on the harmful effects of eating poorly.

In summary, as we go through life it is important to maintain a positive balance so that our cells, tissues, and organs will function properly. If we pay attention to good nutrition (especially with a view to avoiding excess acidity), exercise, and positive emotions, and if we avoid toxic exposure and maximize our innate detoxification systems, then we should be in the healthy zone as illustrated in Figure 2.3. However, if we do not maintain a positive balance, then our cells, tissues, and organs will develop disease, which, if not corrected, will become increasingly serious and lead to premature death.

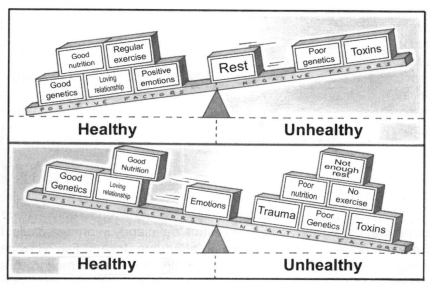

Figure 2.3 TILT Phenomenon

So far I have been painting a rather bleak picture of the dangers lurking in our environment, but don't be discouraged. The good news is that there is real hope of recovery for those who are suffering from chronic health problems as a result of toxicity and bad nutritional habits, as well as for those who want to avoid falling ill as a result of exposure to our contaminated environment. The Cline Medical Centre is one of a growing number of clinics worldwide which specialize in assisting people to recover their health by means of safe, methodically designed programs.[6]

---

[1] Erasmus U. *Fats That Heal Fats That Kill.* Alive Books.1993.

[2] Priority List of Hazardous Substances, U.S. Department of Health and Human Services, www.atsdr.cdc.gov/cercla/05list.html.

[3] Mercury Exposure at High School: BCTF. www.cbc.ca/canada/britishcolumbia/story/2005/11/24/bc_mercury-school20051124.html.

[4] Toxic Nation: A Report on Pollution in Canadians. www.environmentaldefence.ca/reports/toxicnation.

[5] The Importance of an Alkaline Diet, Russell Jaffe, MD, PhD.

[6] The Institute for Functional Medicine (www.ifm.org)

Toxins
What Are They and How Bad Can They Be?

Toxins: The Scope of the Problem

It has now been established that 80-90 percent of all chronic diseases, including cancer, can be linked to toxic exposure and influence.[1] A recent article in the *British Medical Journal* concludes that environmental and lifestyle factors play a major role in human disease and account for approximately 75 percent of all cancers. Clearly, modern industry and technology have improved our general standard of living, but we have paid a heavy price because modern technology and industry also have caused a widespread destruction of ecosystems and the wholesale release of toxicants into our environment.[2] These toxicants are primarily heavy metals and chemicals, which have gradually saturated our water, our food, and the air we breathe. Consequently, we are unable to avoid exposure to toxins that bio-accumulate and bio-concentrate in the food that we have learned to produce so abundantly. Moreover, we remain largely unaware of the presence of these toxins because, for the most part, we cannot see, smell, taste, or feel them. At the Cline Medical Centre, I have carefully taken the histories of thousands of people; remarkably, the large majority of them were unaware of the toxic influences that had in fact harmed their health.

As I pointed out in Chapter 1, our bodies seek balance, a steady state that I compared to a seesaw that might tilt one way or the other depending on how the weight is distributed. The ideal state of equilibrium is sometimes called "homeodynamic balance," and it can be influenced by a number of factors. Thus, on the left side of the seesaw we find positive genetic influences, good nutrition, exercise, healthy emotions, and supportive relationships. On the right side are negative genetic influences, poor nutrition, lack of exercise, negative emotions, various traumas, toxin accumulation and poor or stressful relationships.

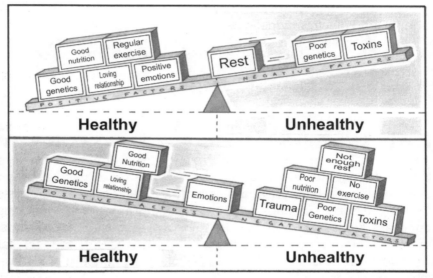

Figure 3.1 TILT Phenomenon

Before we are born, we have already been exposed to many of these influences, which continue to affect us throughout our lives. For instance, even a fetus in the womb can be exposed to the harmful effects of mercury. If the mother consumes fish that is high in mercury, then mercury will accumulate in the developing nervous system of the fetus. If, during pregnancy, the mother has dental work involving the addition of new mercury amalgams or the changing of old amalgams, mercury again will make its way to the fetus. After birth, the baby faces further exposure to mercury in the form of vaccines containing thimerosal as a preservative. Visits to the dentist and the insertion of mercury amalgams into the teeth, as well as the consumption of fish containing mercury, will gradually increase the body's mercury burden. Over a period of many years mercury can accumulate and have a toxic influence on cellular function, even though it might well elude detection. Mercury has been called "the great masquerader", because more than 200 symptoms are associated with this poisonous metal, and it is all too easy to interpret these symptoms as indicating other kinds of disease. Also, for most of us, not just one toxin causes us to be ill, but rather the gradual accumulation of a variety of metals, chemicals, biological agents, and electromagnetic fields, which build up until one day the TILT Phenomenon comes into play. In my clinical practice, I have discovered that there is almost always a "last straw event," such as a car accident, an emotional trauma, or a viral illness, after which the whole system shifts, and a person becomes chronically ill.

Yet the good news is that the TILT Phenomenon can be reversed. One of the greatest joys in my life is seeing the positive changes in broken-down people who initially could scarcely drag themselves into my office. Typically, I begin by taking a detailed history and conducting a physical examination, followed by specific tests to support the hypothesis that toxicants are the main underlying problem. Detoxification programs are then instituted, and in most cases recovery occurs as the balance is tilted back so that cellular health is reestablished. As you read through the cases presented in this book, it is my sincere hope that you will gain new insights into the pervasive dangers of toxicity in our world, why our health might have deteriorated, and what we can do about it.

Toxins: The Two Main Types

Toxin comes from the Latin word "toxicum," which means poison. Toxins that affect us from without are referred to as exogenous, and toxins that affect us from within are endogenous. Examples of exogenous toxins are poisonous metals, persistent organic pollutants, various microbes (bacteria, fungi, and viruses), radiation, and abnormal electromagnetic fields. By contrast, endogenous toxins are produced if our cellular processes do not operate in balance, resulting in the buildup of intermediate by-products which cause harmful effects on brain function or energy production, for example.

Another main source of endogenous toxins is the overgrowth of pathogenic organisms in our intestines. The large bowel contains an ecosystem that requires a delicate balance of organisms. An overgrowth of pathogenic organisms, such as candida or parasites, causes a release of toxic substances that can have adverse effects on cellular function in general. In a later chapter I will discuss the negative impact on our health of toxins released from root canals and jawbone infections, and I will also describe how negative emotions can be harmful to our well-being.

Toxins disrupt cellular function in the following five main ways:

1) Positively charged metallic ions can bind to the negatively charged cell membrane lipids and create structural changes.

2) Free metal ions can attract electrons from other molecules which consequently now lack an electron and become unstable. These unstable molecules are known as "free radicals," and they strip electrons off other molecules in order to regain stability. If this occurs in large chain reactions, the degeneration of cells (and, hence, of tissues and organs) is greatly accelerated.

3) Metallic ions can make their way into the power plants of our cells (these power plants are called "mitochondria"), and they decrease energy production significantly. The chemical reactions in our cells require specialized proteins called enzymes in order to make the reactions go forward. Enzymes, like all cellular components, can be thought of as tiny, intricate machines. If the structural integrity of the enzymes is altered, they will not function properly, and key chemical reactions will either slow down or stop altogether. For instance, within the mitochondria a series of enzymes is involved in electron transfer, a process known as the "electron transport chain." At each point of electron transfer an enzyme is required, but if toxic metals bind to this enzyme, the result is a marked diminishment in energy production in the cells.

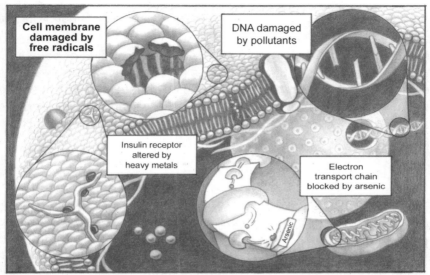

Figure 3.2 Cell Damage

4) Biological toxins are released from organisms in many forms. When released from fungi or yeast, they are called mycotoxins. Likewise, bacteria such as the anaerobic bacteria found in sites of osteonecrosis (dead bone) in the jawbone release highly potent exotoxins. Furthermore, parasites in the intestine release toxins in order to protect themselves from their local environment, and these toxins will poison the person in whose intestines the parasites inhabit. Toxins released from these various organisms can in turn cause structural damage to cell membranes, disrupt enzymes from functioning, and adversely affect DNA (the genetic code). Exotoxins released from root canal treated teeth are especially harmful, as I will show in a later chapter.

5) Persistent organic pollutants, such as pesticides, are carbon-based compounds that are for the most part lipid (fat) soluble. This means that they are attracted to lipid-rich tissues, such as the nervous system. Once these organic toxins gain entrance to a new

cell, they make their way to the nucleus and bind to the DNA. This can potentially cause alteration in the structure and function of the DNA, which can then lead to cancer formation.

In the above five ways in which toxins disrupt cellular function, the end result is that the TILT Phenomenon comes into play as cells lose their ability to tolerate further toxic exposure. Ill health inevitably follows.

A Look Back in History

In order to illustrate the devastatingly lethal effects of heavy metal poisoning, let us for a moment look back to the year 1810.[3] At that time, mercury was a valuable commodity, and large amounts were used to purify gold and silver ores. Mercury was also used in industries such as gilding, plating, mirror-making, and hat manufacturing, and it was prescribed for the treatment of infectious diseases such as syphilis. Spain had virtual control of the mercury market because cinnabar (mercury sulfide) mines were plentiful in Spain as well as in Spanish America. The cinnabar was smelted and made into what was then called "quicksilver" – what we know today as liquid mercury or elemental mercury.

In 1810, Britain, Spain, and Portugal formed an alliance against Napoleon Bonaparte's armies as the French were attempting to gain control of Spain, partly to ensure naval access to the Mediterranean and the Atlantic. On March 4, 1810, a hurricane hit the Spanish port of Cadiz, and the flood surge that followed stranded many Spanish ships close to the French-controlled shore. One of the stranded ships, La Purisima Concepcion, had in its hold a very large shipment of quicksilver originating in South America.

Over several nights, British sailors in longboats were able to remove 130 tons of the liquid mercury, which they placed aboard two ships: the HMS Triumph and the HMS Phipps. The mercury was stored in large leather bladders, which were then placed in iron-hooped strongboxes on the lowest deck of each vessel. Unfortunately, the leather eroded, and many tons of mercury flooded the holds of the two ships. Because mercury was such a precious commodity, many enterprising sailors concealed as much of it as they could.

Over the following weeks, 200 of the 650 men on board the Triumph presented with symptoms of mercury toxicity. These included copious salivation, oral ulcers, partial paralysis, tremors, pulmonary congestion, various bowel complaints, skin eruptions, gum problems, and loss of teeth. The ship's surgeon and purser were among the most severely affected because they bunked beside the mercury storage area. Three men succumbed from pulmonary disease and two from facial gangrene. All the animals on the ship died.

The Triumph was thoroughly cleaned several times, and 8000 pounds of mercury-contaminated biscuits were thrown out. Even so, a fine metallic powder continued to accumulate, and on the ship's next voyage in June 1810, forty-four sailors became seriously ill. The ship's surgeon, Henry Plowman, correctly deduced that mercuric vapors were affecting the crew. He ordered increased ventilation to the lower deck, and no further cases of mercury poisoning occurred; nevertheless, the ship never sailed again. An eyewitness to these distressing events drew a straightforward conclusion: "Conversing with several officers of the British Navy on the subject, I was induced to believe that the accident proceeded altogether from the ignorance of all those concerned." From the outset, ignorance about the effects of mercury and its lethal vapor was indeed chiefly to blame for the catastrophe.

This historical event illustrates how seriously health can be altered and even destroyed because of toxic exposure. Of course, most people who come to my clinic have not had such a severe and acute exposure as the sailors on board the Triumph. Nonetheless, the vast majority of my patients have had ongoing, low-level exposure to toxic substances, and over many years such exposure can produce results not dissimilar to those experienced by the unfortunate sailors.

After reading stories such as the historical account above, many of you might think, "It could never happen to me." But, sadly, it could, and I will end this section with a little anecdote. I admit that I am a fan of James Bond movies, and I have often thought that the Russian character Boris in *Golden Eye* is pertinent to my professional interests. Boris was the ultimate computer nerd working as a programmer for a secret Russian installation. Whenever he was triumphant in hacking into a heavily fortified program, he would stand up, lift his arms, and proclaim, "I am inveencable!" At the end of the show, he does this one last time and immediately dies after being suddenly immersed in liquid nitrogen. We might be more like Boris than we think, especially if we persist in denying our vulnerability to the toxic influences I have been describing. Let me now introduce you to Josh.

Josh's Case

When I first saw Josh in the waiting room of my clinic, he was sitting on the floor in a corner. He was very well muscled, dressed in leather, with a red bandana around his head. He was talking quite loudly, and I admit to being a bit nervous as I led him into the examining room.

At the time, Josh was thirty-six years old. He had been a construction worker, a housepainter, and an auto-body worker. At eighteen, he had experienced what sounded like a severe viral illness with a high fever, fatigue, severe muscle pain, sweating, and headaches. He was quite ill for approximately three months, after which the muscle and joint pains migrated throughout his body. In his various jobs, he had been exposed to several heavy metals and chemicals. Additionally, during his childhood he began getting mercury amalgams (silver fillings), and these had all been removed and replaced with further mercury amalgams. He also had a number of gold crowns interspersed amongst his fillings. Josh told me that for many years severe fatigue had prevented him from working. His sleep was interrupted, and he awoke each morning feeling unrefreshed.

When he was thirty years old, Josh was admitted to a hospital for three months, suffering from severe depression and psychosis. During the next six years, he was readmitted to the psychiatric unit several times. There was no family history of mental illness, and a large number of medications were tried, including antidepressants, antipsychotics, tranquilizers, and sedatives, but these brought about very little improvement. Josh also had recurrent ulcers in his mouth, chronically swollen gums, a burning sensation in his tongue, and a constant metallic taste. His short-term memory was not as sharp as it had been, and he admitted to erectile dysfunction. He denied any use of street drugs and he consumed alcohol only occasionally. His speech was quite animated, and he jumped erratically from topic to topic. Several times during the interview he asked me if I would prescribe gold for him to take orally. (Josh is the only person who has ever made this request, and I interpreted it as a delusion he was having).

On examining him, I found Josh's blood pressure was elevated at 170/104. He had thirteen mercury amalgams, two gold crowns, and one porcelain crown present. He demonstrated an exaggerated response to painful stimuli, and all eighteen tender points for fibromyalgia were positive. His neurological examination was within normal limits, as was his blood work. I then performed a DMPS challenge test[4], which revealed elevated mercury (89 mcg, with normal less than 3), lead (20 mcg, with normal less than 15), and tin (14 mcg, with normal less than 6). (see Figure 3.3) Josh's mercury level is especially significant because a reading of 50 or greater is considered proof of toxicity.

Doctor's Data, Inc.
P.O. Box 111
West Chicago, Illinois 60186-0111
CALL TOLL FREE (800) 323-2784
Fax: (630) 231-9190
E-mail: inquiries@doctorsdata.com
Web site: www.doctorsdata.com

James T. Hicks, M.D., Ph.D., FCAP
Medical Director
CLIA ID # 14D0646670, Medicare Provider # 548453

ELEMENTS REGARDED AS TOXIC

Elements	Per gram Creatinine Result (µg/g creatinine)	Reference Range* (µg/g creatinine)	Within Ref. Range	Elevated	Very Elevated
Aluminum	< dl	0 - 35			
Antimony	.4	0 - 5	•		
Arsenic	27	0 - 100	••••		
Beryllium	< dl	0 - .5			
Bismuth	2.1	0 - 30	•		
Cadmium	.4	0 - 3	•••		
Lead	20	0 - 15	••••••••••••••••••		
Mercury	89	0 - 3	••••••••••••••••••••••••••••••••••••	••••••••	••••••••••••••••••
Nickel	4.3	0 - 12	•••••		
Platinum	< dl	0 - 2			
Thallium	.1	0 - 14	•		
Thorium	< dl	0 - 12			
Tin	14	0 - 6	••••••••••••••••••••••		
Tungsten	0	0 - 23	•		
Uranium	< dl	0 - 1			

OTHER TESTS

	Result (mg/dl)	Reference Range (mg/dl)	2 SD Low	1 SD Low	MEAN	1 SD High	2 SD High
Creatinine	195	75 - 200			•••••••••••	••••••	

Methodology: Analyzed by Induction Coupled Plasma Mass Spectrometry (ICP-MS). Creatinine by Jaffe method. "dl"=detection limit. *No safe levels established.	Comments: (Post provocative challenge.) hg checked

Figure 3.3

Josh then went through a mercury and heavy metal detoxification program at our clinic. This program included attention to diet, a regimen of supplements, once-a-month injections of DMPS, and careful extraction of his mercury amalgams. An intravenous infusion of vitamins and minerals was given the day following the DMPS injection and dental work.

Josh reported that in the week following the DMPS injection, his energy increased significantly, and after his third treatment he felt so much better that he was able to paint the outside of his girlfriend's house. Following his fourth treatment, he had no further muscle pain, his mind was clear, and his energy had increased significantly. By and by, he was able to return to the workforce.

Case Discussion

It is useful to think about this case in terms of the TILT Phenomenon. Josh's toxic exposure began in childhood with the placement of mercury amalgams in his teeth. At one point, these amalgams were replaced with yet more mercury, and his toxic load was further increased with each house he painted and each car he refinished. At eighteen, he had what sounded like a severe viral illness or exposure to an unknown microbe. This was the key event that tipped the balance, and in order for his health to be restored, these accumulated toxic foci had to be removed patiently and gradually.

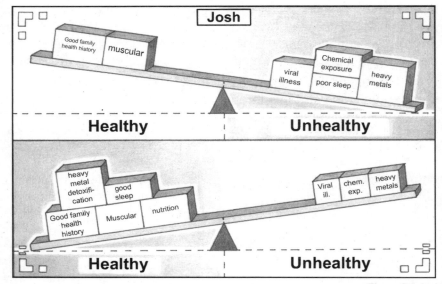

Figure 3.4 Josh

Like Josh, if we are not good at detoxifying ourselves, and if we are not careful about how we live, then a last-straw event will likely occur, and our whole system will TILT for the worse. I would like to end this chapter by giving the last word to Merrill Garnett, DDS, PhD, a brilliant cancer researcher. In his book, *First Pulse*[5], he describes in some arresting verses how external agents influence us whether we are aware of them or not:

> The external intrudes continuously.
> It intrudes in plasma. It intrudes in blood.
> It not only intrudes on the outside of the cell,
> but comes into us at the most
> intimate levels of information transfer.
> It twists and turns and makes things grow differently.
> We are not insulated. We are not isolated.
> We are an open window to nature.

The external is all through us. It structures us.
Problems arise because of our denial of this fact.

We typically see the organism as a defined entity.
But, we are fashioned of the universe, and the
universe streams through us.
The universe, the external, is an onslaught and
an interaction which modifies and selects at the
cellular and molecular continuously.

If we choose to understand these events that
make us one with the universe,
We can then avoid certain changes that cause disease
and untimely death.

---

[1] Sharpe RM, Irvine DS. How strong is the evidence of a link between environmental chemicals and adverse effects on human reproductive health? BMJ. 2004 Feb 21. 328(7437):447-51.

[2] United Nations Environment Program (UNEP), One Planet Many People: Atlas of our Changing Environment. June 2005.

[3] Doherty MJ. The quicksilver prize. Mercury vapor poisoning aboard HMS Triumph and HMS Phipps. Neurology Volume 62 • Number 6 • March 23, 2004.

[4] DMPS stands for 2,3,-**Di**mercapto-**p**ropane-1-**s**ulfonic acid, a chelating agent that binds many heavy metals forming stable complexes, which are excreted through the kidneys into the urine. After an injection, urine is collected and sent to a toxicology laboratory where quantitative analysis for heavy metals is performed.

[5] Garnett M, et al. (2001) *First pulse: a Personal Journey in Cancer Research*, 2nd Ed., First Pulse Projects Inc., New York.

Basic Toxicology and Functional Toxicology

Toxicology

The term toxicology means "the study of toxins," and it describes a field of medicine and research that assesses the effects of toxins on populations. One problem is that broad conclusions about the effect of toxins on a population do not necessarily reflect the actual dangers to which people are exposed. A prime example is how lead toxicity was defined by the Center for Disease Control and Prevention (CDCP) over the past several decades.

During the 1960s, the diagnosis of lead toxicity was made if a person's whole blood lead level was 60 mcg/dl (micrograms per deciliter) or higher. This meant that people with levels below 60 were not considered to have a significant amount of lead present, and certainly not enough to treat. By 1975 the CDCP deemed that a better level would be 35 mcg/dl. In 1985 the level was lowered to 25 mcg/dl, and again in 1991 it was further decreased to 10 mcg/dl. These changes mean that many more people are now diagnosed with lead toxicity, confirming the seriousness of the problem. In April 2003, the *New England Journal of Medicine*[1] published a landmark article demonstrating that with each 10 mcg rise in blood lead level, a child's IQ falls by 4.6 points. Even more startling is the fact that for blood lead levels between 1 and 10 mcg, the IQ falls by 7.4 points. The conclusion that even low levels of lead are inversely associated with IQ scores confirms that many more children are seriously affected by lead than was previously thought. Even the 10 mcg threshold is now questioned in face of a growing, widespread recognition that there is no safe level of lead for humans.

In an excellent article, M. Shea MD, MPH,[2] challenges a widely held principle among toxicologists that "the presence of a chemical in the blood or urine does not necessarily mean a person is at risk for adverse health effects." Dr. Shea also challenges the concept that "the dose makes the poison" (that is, whether or not you will be poisoned depends on how large a dose you take). Instead, Dr. Shea argues that low-dose exposure is not necessarily safe exposure, and although the claim that "the dose makes the poison" may be true for adults (although this also is questionable), it simply cannot be applied to rapidly developing, growing children. The timing, pattern, and amount of exposure may be as important in determining health outcomes as the fact that the exposure occurred.

For example, lead, mercury, and PCBs (polychlorinated biphenyls) are known to be toxic to the developing brain of a fetus and of a young child at exposures that would not adversely affect a pregnant woman or other adults. Recent studies on lead toxicity suggest that no level of exposure is safe for the developing nervous system. Indeed, exposure of the developing brain to methylmercury early in pregnancy leads to permanent alteration of the brain's architecture. This dire consequence can be related to something as routine as the consumption of fish in early pregnancy.

A growing number of similar examples teach us that it is dangerous to assume that general guidelines are reliable in all cases and that "low-dose" exposures are safe. In short, it is important to realize that "no evidence of harm is not equivalent to evidence of no harm." As Dr. Shea says:

"Our habits of linear thinking have trained us well in the one-cause/one-disease model of illness, but the likelihood of developing clinical illness is modulated by multiple factors including nutritional status, age, lifestyle, and many others. This is certainly true for environmental illness. For the well-characterized environmental exposures such as lead, mercury, and some pesticides, we have found that when exposed, children often acquire higher internal doses than adults, toxicity occurs at lower levels than anticipated compared with adults, and lifelong toxicity to critical systems during development occur in ways unparalleled by adult exposures."

Functional Medicine and Functional Toxicology

Functional medicine is a new field of healthcare that focuses especially on each person as an individual.[3] Functional toxicology has developed within this broader field, and it differs from traditional toxicology in that it examines and treats chronic, sublethal, and often subclinical toxicological factors that impair physiological, emotional, and physical function. The physician practicing functional medicine recognizes that people are unique in their ability to detoxify and that general guidelines about safe levels of toxins do not always describe the experience of individual people. For instance, if an individual has impaired detoxification abilities, even small amounts of a toxin can have a large negative impact at the cellular level. But if an individual has excellent detoxification abilities, toxic substances will be removed and excreted from the body without harm. In short, functional toxicology takes seriously Dr. Shea's challenge of the idea that "the dose makes the poison," as well as her recommendation that we consider how "multiple factors" might contribute to an illness. The following eight key points are especially important to consider when we deal with detoxification from the perspective of functional medicine.

1.) Genetic Limitations in Detoxification Ability. In earlier periods of human history, most chemicals and drugs to which we are now exposed did not exist. In general, our systems of detoxification and elimination were not required to deal with the tens of thousands of biologically persistent chemicals to which we are now exposed each day. Our detoxification systems have had to adapt to the seriously increased stresses and challenges presented by modern life, and, not surprisingly, we differ in our ability to deal effectively with the new toxicants. New methods of testing can now predict an individual's ability to detoxify and can allow the practitioner to pinpoint which detoxification mechanisms are malfunctioning.[4]

2.) Genetic Predisposition to Toxin-Related Illnesses. Many people have either genetic mutations or single nucleotide polymorphisms, also known as SNPs or "snips." These are genetic variations that occur when a single nucleotide substitution is made in the DNA sequence. This kind of substitution can result in alterations in the way that proteins are produced in the cell, so that the ability of the individual to detoxify is altered. SNPs account for 90 percent of all the human genetic variations which predispose us to the development of certain illnesses. Examples include cancer, autoimmune disorders such as rheumatoid arthritis, and the autistic spectrum disorders. We should take note that not all children who are exposed to metal and chemical toxicants go on to develop autism. However, those who are genetically predisposed not to eliminate toxins effectively will often develop these types of disorders. The same holds true for Alzheimer's in adults. Consequently, we need to attend carefully to each individual person's genetic predispositions as a key to preventing the onset of disease.

3.) Toxic Exposure. It is important to identify the quantity, intensity, duration, and diversity of exposure to toxic substances. When taking a patient's history I often have to enquire closely about past exposure to toxicants because people frequently forget or do not realize that they have been at risk. As we have seen, in most cases no single toxin is the culprit but rather a range of metals, organic chemicals, and biological toxins to which individuals previously have been exposed.

4.) The Minimization of Toxic Exposure. At the start of the detoxification process it is important to minimize further exposure to the toxicants at which treatment is aimed. For example, patients with high levels of mercury will sometimes ask me if they can go ahead with a detoxification program without getting the mercury amalgams removed from their teeth. I explain that mercury amalgams in the teeth constantly off-gas, and it does not make sense to take mercury out of the body if a constant stream of mercury is going back in. The same principle applies to all kinds of toxic exposure.

5.) Diet and Antioxidant Status. For most of us, a major exposure to toxins occurs through the food we eat. I find that most people who are chronically ill are nutritionally deficient and are not getting optimal macronutrients such as protein, good fats, and proper carbohydrates. As well, they are lacking the micronutrients required in the thousands of ongoing chemical reactions in our cells. Simple changes in diet and the addition of key nutritional supplements can often assist in laying a foundation that will enable the person to detoxify and eliminate properly.

6.) Gastrointestinal Health. The surface area of the gastrointestinal tract is the largest interface we have with the external world. It has been estimated that the size of this surface is the equivalent of a collegiate basketball court. Also, the gastrointestinal tract (with its associated organs – the liver, gallbladder, and pancreas) is a major system that enables detoxification and elimination. Consequently, failure to correct any dysfunction in this important system before detoxification efforts are started can lead to a worsening of the patient's health.

7.) Exercise. Most of us in North America do not exercise sufficiently, but I find that people who are chronically ill tend to exercise very little, if at all. In order to facilitate detoxification and elimination, I always encourage my patients to exercise daily.

8.) Ongoing Detoxification. Often patients think that once they have finished a detoxification treatment program and are feeling well again, the detoxification process is complete. But when I am asked how often we should detoxify, my answer is, "Daily." If we do not pay attention to keeping our detoxification systems working well, the toxic load will gradually build up again.

To conclude this section, I would like to cite Sidney Baker, MD, who amusingly but seriously introduces us to what he calls the "Tack Principle[5]." Dr. Baker asks us to consider what we would do if a patient complains of pain in the buttocks, and we observe three tacks sticking into the patient's rear end.

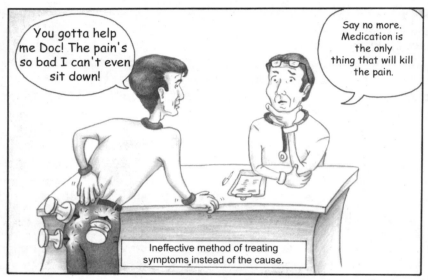

Figure 4.1 Ineffective Method of Treating Symptoms Instead of the Cause

a) We prescribe ASA, acetaminophen or a painkiller and send the patient home.

b) We tell the patient that there are no such things as tacks and the pain is imaginary.

c) We explain that some researchers believe that tacks exist and are conducting preliminary trials, but it will be years before any definitive treatment exists.

d) We recognize that tacks are the problem, and we remove them.

The fact is, Dr. Baker's tacks do exist in the form of toxins, and it is often quite obvious that this is the case even though the plain truth is frequently unrecognized. Once we allow ourselves to acknowledge the tacks, the eight guidelines I have listed above can provide an effective approach to removing the real source of the problem.

---

[1] Canfield RL, Henderson CR, Cory-Slechta DA, Cox C, Jusko TA, Lanphear BP, et al. Intellectual impairment in children with blood lead concentrations below 10 micrograms per deciliter. N Engl J Med 2003; 348:1517-26.

[2] Shea KM. Protecting our children from environmental hazards in the face of limited data-a precautionary approach is needed. J Pediatr. 2004 Aug; 145(2): 145-7.

[3] The Textbook of Functional Medicine 2006. www.functionalmedicine.org

[4] www.genovations.com

[5] *Detoxification & Healing: The Key to Optimal Health,* Sidney M. Baker MD, Keats Pub, Inc. 1997.

Toxins - How to Deal with Them

Although it is important for us to understand the basic concepts of toxicology and to realize what a toxic a world we live in, it is also important to understand how we ourselves are designed to deal with toxins. Practitioners of functional medicine can provide assistance to rid us of accumulated toxins, but if we did not have innate abilities to prevent the absorption of toxins and to rid ourselves of them, our lives would be very short indeed. Therefore, in this chapter we will discuss the central importance of a healthy gastrointestinal system and the role that food choices play within this system. Then we will briefly consider the other detoxification organs that each of us possesses.

The Gastrointestinal Tract: The Key to Healthy Living

The gastrointestinal (GI) system is basically a tube from the mouth to the anus, approximately twenty-seven feet long. It is organized into a number of segments from the mouth and esophagus to the stomach, the small intestine, and the large intestine, ending at the anus. The passage within this tube, or tract, is considered to be outside the body (see Figure 5.1). At first glance this does not make sense – how can the inside of our gastrointestinal tract be considered outside the body? The answer is actually quite simple. The gastrointestinal tract has an opening (orifice) to the outside world at each end – the mouth at the top and the anus at the bottom. If both of these orifices were held open and if air were used to inflate the tube, you can see how it really is like a long balloon within our bodies.

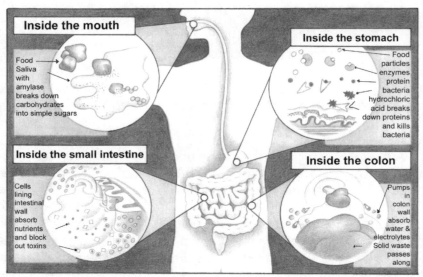

Figure 5.1 The Gastrointestinal Tract

This is a very important concept to grasp, because it explains not only how the gastrointestinal tract is the largest surface area we have with the external world, but also why its highly complex operations have far-reaching effects on our health.

Within the gastrointestinal tract, our food is broken down, digested, and made into a liquid that passes over the large surface area where nutrients are absorbed, harmful substances are kept out, and waste products are excreted. When we first see or smell food, signals go to specialized cells in the lining of the stomach which secrete hydrochloric acid and certain enzymes that break the food down into components that can be absorbed. For example, when we first begin to chew our food, various glands in the mouth secrete saliva. The saliva contains an enzyme called amylase, which breaks down carbohydrates (carbon-based compounds such as fruits, vegetables, and starches) into simple sugars.

Once food is swallowed it enters the stomach, where hydrochloric acid, mucus, and various enzymes are added. The food is then held in the stomach for a period of time and churned, much as a washing machine churns clothes. In this process, hydrochloric acid serves two main purposes. First, it initiates the breakdown of protein (from beef, poultry, fish, dairy, legumes, and so on) into amino acids. Second, it kills bacteria present in our food (especially raw food). Hydrochloric acid, therefore, is vital both for digestion and protection.

After our food is liquefied in the stomach, it is slowly released into the first part of the small intestine. The upper part of the small intestine, the duodenum, has several important organs attached to it: the liver, the gallbladder, and the pancreas. When food is in the stomach, hormonal signals tell the liver, gallbladder, and pancreas to begin releasing bile and pancreatic fluid into the small intestine in preparation for the liquid food that is coming down the pipe, so to speak. Pancreatic secretions are rich in enzymes such as amylase (which breaks down carbohydrates into simple sugars), proteases (which break down protein into amino acids), and lipases (which break fat down into fatty acids). The pancreatic secretions are also highly alkaline, thereby counteracting the acidic liquid coming from the stomach. The bile contains bile acids, which assist in the absorption of fatty acids, and it also contains toxins that have been excreted from the liver.

Our liquid food now begins the long journey down the twenty-two feet of small intestine and across the large surface area where nutrients are absorbed. The millions of cells lining the intestinal surface must be functioning well so that maximum absorption of nutrients occurs and toxic substances are kept out. If the integrity of this surface is disturbed, then proper absorption will not take place. Things that can disrupt the integrity of the surface include the consumption of foods that produce allergic reactions, toxic substances in the foods (such as heavy metals, pesticides, and alcohol), the consumption of foods that are lacking in nutrients, and the overgrowth of pathogenic microbes (such as various kinds of yeasts, parasites, and bacteria). Also, if the cells lining the intestine become injured, inflammation and swelling can occur, and a number of adverse effects will result. For instance, partially digested food particles and toxic substances can cross the lining of the intestine (this is known as "leaky gut") and stimulate the local immune system, possibly causing local and systemic inflammatory reactions.

In addition, the surface area for the absorption of nutrients can substantially decrease. In people suffering with celiac disease (the inflammatory destruction of the lining of the intestine due to reactions from the consumption of gluten), the surface area can be as small as a tennis court, compared to the normal equivalent of a basketball court, in which case most of the nutrients supplied by food are not absorbed. Finally, undigested food sitting in the intestine can cause microbes such as yeast and bacteria to grow excessively. These organisms then secrete noxious substances such as alcohol and ketones, as well as substances that can activate the immune system and increase inflammation throughout the body. People suffering from this problem often tell me that after consuming food they develop abdominal bloating, cramps, cognitive changes (for instance, they feel as if they are drunk), headaches, and muscle or joint pain.

Everything that is absorbed from the intestine ends up in a series of veins leading to the liver. The blood in these veins contains nutrients, partially digested food, immune complexes, as well as highly toxic substances that have to be processed by the liver before entering the general circulation. The leftovers from the liquid food, secreted toxins, and the shed lining of the small intestine (this lining is renewed rapidly and sheds frequently, much like our skin) then enters the large intestine or colon, which is approximately three feet long. The colon has a number of functions, the first of which is the absorption of water from liquid feces. Some experts have estimated that there are far more organisms in our colon then there are cells in our bodies. If each of us has approximately

40 trillion cells, this would translate into approximately 100 trillion organisms in the colon, constituting an important ecosystem for us to maintain. Unfortunately, because of poor dietary choices and the overgrowth of pathogenic organisms, the colon becomes a war zone where pathogenic organisms struggle to win the upper hand. If they succeed, the result is that various yeast forms, parasites, and even bacteria invade the body. Overgrowth of such organisms can in turn result in the secretion of multitudes of toxic and noxious substances that enter our systems, producing widespread cellular dysfunction. However, it should also be mentioned that many "friendly" organisms in the colon produce beneficial substances, such as certain B vitamins.

A variety of signs and symptoms can be linked to gastrointestinal dysfunction. Some of these are bad breath, coated tongue, dry flaky skin, brittle hair, dilated blood vessels in the cheeks and nose, rashes, nasal congestion, frequent and recurrent infections, muscle or joint pain, headaches, depression or anxiety, cognitive dysfunction, and fatigue. Also, many medical conditions can be linked directly or indirectly to gastrointestinal dysfunction, including acne rosacea, alcoholism, autism, celiac disease, childhood ear infections, chronic yeast infections, chronic fatigue syndrome, colitis, Crohn's disease, dermatitis herpetiformis (associated with celiac disease), diverticulitis, eczema, fibromyalgia, gastritis, hemorrhoids, irritable bowel syndrome, liver dysfunction, migraine headaches, multiple chemical sensitivities, peptic ulcer disease, helicobacter pylori infection, pernicious anemia, psoriasis, rheumatoid arthritis, ulcerative colitis, and urticaria (hives),

Let Food Be Your Medicine

I have described the gastrointestinal system in some detail because its workings are so important to good health. The simple truth is that without proper food we will perish, and the wonderful complexities by which the gastrointestinal tract supplies us with nourishment are vulnerable to a wide variety of toxins that can compromise its efficiency. But although we require a healthy gastrointestinal system to assimilate nutrients, it is also the case that the food we decide to eat can affect our gastrointestinal health. The ancient Greek physician, Hippocrates, speaks wisely when he says, "Let food be your medicine and medicine your food." If we can obtain high-quality food that we are able to digest and assimilate properly, there is no better source of micronutrients for our bodies. Unfortunately, however, much of the food that we consume is grown in soil that has been depleted of nutrients, such as trace minerals. If these minerals are not present in the soil, plants cannot manufacture them. Also, soil is frequently contaminated by herbicides, pesticides, and insecticides, and there are even places in the world where DDT is still in use. If we consume food produced in such environments, the contaminating chemicals end up inside us, and unless we are good at detoxifying, the levels of these chemicals will build up. Furthermore, certain toxic substances such as a heavy metals and persistent organic pollutants can bioaccumulate in the food chain, resulting in high concentrations of toxins in various meats and fish.

Again, processed foods often contain substances that are foreign to our bodies. A well-known example is the alteration of fats in order to increase their shelf life. Hydrogenation (a process whereby hydrogen is added to oils or fats to make them solid or semisolid at room temperature) does indeed improve the texture of baked goods and increases the shelf life of food, but it also alters the chemical bond structure of the fats and produces what are known as trans fatty acids. Trans fats are altered forms of fat that are foreign to our bodies, and when inserted into cell membranes, they can make the membranes more rigid and less fluid. Cell membrane components, such as proteins, also are adversely affected, and cell function is therefore impaired. For further discussion of this topic, please see Appendix A.

Food Allergies and Intolerances

Based on observing thousands of patients, I have come to conclude that almost everyone suffers from either true food allergies or intolerances of certain foods. This unsettling conclusion reflects the fact that the processes of digestion and assimilation are individual, and not all foods are equally good for all people. But it also suggests that our gastrointestinal tracts are not able to handle our increasingly contaminated sources of nourishment.

Food allergies are characterized by reactions mediated through the immune system, and these reactions can be immediate and sometimes life threatening. For instance, when people who are highly allergic to peanuts are exposed to even the smell of peanuts, they can develop immediate swelling of the skin (hives) or a more serious swelling of the mouth, throat, and membranes in the lungs and intestines. Most allergic reactions to foods are not so dramatic, but are often delayed by several hours or even one or two days.

Food intolerances (as distinct from allergies), on the other hand, are characterized by reactions to nontoxic substances within the foods. A fairly common example is intolerance to the milk sugar called lactose. People who have this problem are not able to break lactose down into simple sugars that can be absorbed across the gastrointestinal wall. Therefore, lactose remains in the intestine and becomes food for bacteria that convert it into hydrogen and methane gases, which then cause bloating. Undigested lactose can also cause diarrhea and cramps.

There is good and reliable testing for immediate, life-threatening food allergies. Basically, a blood test looks for evidence of an immunoglobulin called IgE, and the test is both easy to do and accurate. Skin-prick testing is not reliable for food allergies, but blood tests are available that will detect delayed types of allergic food reactions. These blood tests are more reliable than skin testing, but they are expensive and must be interpreted with close attention to the patient's symptoms. One such test is the Lymphocyte Response Assay developed by Russell Jaffe, MD, PhD. This test is generally effective and detects sensitivities to foods and to many toxins we discuss in this book.[1] Some practitioners also use Autonomic Response Testing, which uses muscle testing through biofeedback of the autonomic nervous system to determine disturbances in the body and to suggest potential remedies. The results are not entirely reliable, because it is frequently difficult to eliminate bias on the part of the practitioner, the patient, or both.

The most reliable way to test for delayed food reactions is a properly conducted food elimination diet. This involves removing a large number of foods from the diet all at once. The GI system then has an extended break, allowing the lining of the intestine to heal. After approximately four weeks, the prohibited foods are reintroduced one group at a time every four days, and the person is instructed to notice any unusual symptoms that may occur. The details of this approach are described in Appendix B, at the end of this book. In our clinic, we have found this to be a very useful exercise, as well as a simple and inexpensive way to improve health relatively quickly. It also prepares our chronically ill patients for further, more challenging detoxification.

Several years ago, my friend and colleague, Michael Lyon, MD, and I conducted a research project on the food elimination diet. The project involved working with a group of seventy children with Attention Deficit Hyperactivity Disorder. These seventy children were randomly split into three groups. One group acted as a control, the second group was placed on an elimination diet, and the third group was placed on an elimination diet supplemented by a medical food product. My eldest daughter was in the second group. At the time, she was fourteen years old, overweight, with a C average in school. She had troubles with self-esteem and also suffered with allergic rhinitis and asthma. She often complained of abdominal bloating and cramps. She was diagnosed with the inattentive form of ADHD, which meant that often her mind would be off in space.

We observed that the vast majority of the children in the elimination diet groups displayed remarkable improvements in their behaviors and attentiveness. When the offending foods were reintroduced one at a time every four days, the children's behaviors deteriorated, sometimes within one hour, but usually within one day. My daughter certainly experienced an outstanding improvement not only in her attentiveness, but also in her general quality of life. Her attentiveness improved so significantly that her academic grades increased to mostly As and Bs. She lost a significant amount of weight, and she found that her emotions were more stable, without the mood swings she had previously experienced. Her allergy symptoms also improved significantly, as did her self-esteem and confidence. Towards the end of the study, she had a birthday party and "pigged out" on the foods that she used to consume, such as cake, chips, pop, and ice cream. The next day, she had abdominal bloating and cramps, she became very emotional, and her nasal passages were congested. The wonderful thing was that she herself made the connection between the consumption of wheat, sugar, and diary products and the resulting unpleasant symptoms. She has been much healthier since making this connection and adjusting her diet accordingly. Recently, she graduated with distinction from the Costume Studies program at Dalhousie University in Nova Scotia, Canada. (I apologize for bragging.)

The knowledge that I gained from this research project I now apply regularly to patients who come to my clinic, and sometimes I find that the elimination of offending foods and the addition of healthy foods is the only intervention required to restore good health. Often further steps need to be taken, but adjusting a person's diet provides a foundation on which we can build if we decide to use other detoxification techniques.

To further illustrate the importance in dealing with gastrointestinal issues when attempting to detoxify, I will now introduce you to Daniel.

Daniel's Case

Daniel, a forty-seven-year-old schoolteacher, was diagnosed with chronic fatigue syndrome at age thirty-three. Although his energy was significantly depleted, Daniel was still able to teach at that time. Besides trying several other therapies, he had read about the mercury amalgam (silver filling) debate, and when he was thirty-eight years old, he decided to get his amalgams changed. He had approximately fifteen mercury amalgams, and his dentist removed them in one sitting. Following this, his health declined precipitously to the point where he had to take one year off from teaching. In short, the sudden and significant exposure to mercury from the dental work resulted in a negative tipping point that plunged him into ill health. He developed sensitivities to chemicals, severe fatigue, severe sleep disturbances, outbreaks on his skin, headaches, and "brain fog."

At forty-three years old, Daniel began working with a biological dentist who found several cavitations (cavitations, or osteonecrosis, are areas of diseased or dead bone in the jaw and are further described in Chapter 12 – "Our Toxic Mouths"). These cavitations were treated, and extensive neural therapy was done (this procedure is described in the chapter "Electromagnetic Fields Can Be Hazardous to Your Health"). One year before I met him, Daniel had seen another physician who administered intravenous DMPS, which is the number-one chelating agent for mercury and other metals. However, the DMPS was administered too quickly, over approximately two minutes. Daniel told me the procedure caused his "kidneys to hurt," and after his treatments he felt much worse for several weeks. Nonetheless, his energy slowly began to improve, and he was able to participate to a limited extent in sports like skiing, basketball, and volleyball. His sleep was much better, but his cognitive functions were still not as clear as they should have been.

Throughout his life, Daniel had an extensive number of operations, including repair of his bilateral pelvis and femur fractures, which occurred at two years old when he was run over by a car. At fifteen years old, he fractured a leg, and at sixteen, he had a tonsillectomy. At twenty-seven, he had surgery on his left shoulder, and at thirty-two, his left leg was shortened. At thirty-two, he also underwent a hemorrhoidectomy, and two years earlier he had endured several episodes of prostatitis. Daniel also had childhood sexual abuse issues, which had been dealt with through extensive counseling.

In his previous occupation as a heavy-duty diesel mechanic, Daniel had several years of exposure to chemical substances, and for many years he had symptoms of dysbiosis (disordered gastrointestinal function), including bloating after he ate, and alternating constipation and diarrhea. On closer questioning, I learned that in his mid-twenties he had been incarcerated in a prison in Morocco for two months. During that time, he had constant, severe diarrhea that almost killed him. He told me that his gastrointestinal function had never fully recovered, and that he had tried various herbal cleansing programs with little success.

When I examined him, Daniel appeared well, but very thin. He had an upper dental plate and lower partial plate, but his examination was otherwise unremarkable. His CBC (complete blood count), complete blood chemistries, stool testing, and urinalysis were all within normal limits. A DMPS challenge test, completed prior to attending our clinic, revealed elevated mercury (35 mcg, with normal less than 3), but other metals were within reference range. (see Figure 5.2)

Because of Daniel's history of dysentery and ongoing bowel symptoms, and despite the fact that his stool tests were negative, I elected to place him on a three-week course of iodoquinol: 650 mg taken three times daily over twenty days. This is a very old antiparasitic medication. Following this, he had a marked

DETOXIFY FOR LIFE

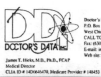

Doctor's Data, Inc.
P.O. Box 111
West Chicago, Illinois 60186-0111
CALL TOLL FREE (800) 323-2784
Fax: (630) 587-7860
E-mail: inquiries@doctorsdata.com
Web site: www.doctorsdata.com

James T. Hicks, M.D., Ph.D., FCAP
Medical Director
CLIA ID # 14D0646470, Medicare Provider # 148453

		DMPS 250MG
Urine Toxic Elements	Lab #:	T
Patient:	Age:	Sex: Male
Doctor:	Acct #:	
c/o:	Collection Type: Random	
Collection Date:	Time:	
Date In: 18 Feb 2000	Date Out: 22 Feb 2000	

ELEMENTS REGARDED AS TOXIC

Elements	Per gram Creatinine Result (µg/g creatinine)	Reference Range* (µg/g creatinine)	Within Ref. Range	Elevated	Very Elevated
Aluminum	< dl	0 - 35			
Antimony	.2	0 - 5	•		
Arsenic	100	0 - 100	•••••••••••••••		
Beryllium	< dl	0 - .5			
Bismuth	< dl	0 - 30			
Cadmium	.9	0 - 2	••••••		✓
Lead	4.4	0 - 15	••••		
Mercury	35	0 - 3	•••••••••••••••	••••••••••••••••••••••••	•••••••
Nickel	3	0 - 12	•••		
Platinum	< dl	0 - 2			
Thallium	.2	0 - 14	•		
Thorium	< dl	0 - 12			
Tin	3	0 - 6	••••••••		
Tungsten	< dl	0 - 23			
Uranium	< dl	0 - 1			

OTHER TESTS

	Result (mg/dl)	Reference Range (mg/dl)	2 SD Low	I SD Low	MEAN	I SD High	2 SD High
Creatinine	28.6	75 - 200	•••••••••••••••••••••				

Methodology: Analyzed by Induction Coupled Plasma Mass Spectrometry (ICP-MS). Creatinine by Jaffe method.

"dl"=detection limit.
*No safe levels established.

Comments:
(Post provocative challenge.)

Figure 5.2

Doctor's Data, Inc.
P.O. Box 111
West Chicago, Illinois 60186-0111
CALL TOLL FREE (800) 323-2784
Fax: (630) 587-7850
E-mail: inquiries@doctorsdata.com
Web site: www.doctorsdata.com

James T. Hicks, M.D., Ph.D., FCAP
Medical Director
CLIA ID # 14D0646470, Medicare Provider # 148453

Urine Toxic Elements

DMPS 4.5 M

Lab #:		
Patient:	Age: 47	Sex: Male
Doctor: John Cline, MD	Acct #: 22580	
c/o: Oceanside Medical Clinic	Collection Type: Random	
Collection Date: 10 Jan 2001	Time:	
Date In: 16 Jan 2001	Date Out: 17 Jan 2001	

ELEMENTS REGARDED AS TOXIC

Elements	Per gram Creatinine Result (µg/g creatinine)	Reference Range* (µg/g creatinine)	Within Ref. Range	Elevated	Very Elevated
Aluminum	< dl	0 - 35			
Antimony	1.8	0 - 5	•••••		
Arsenic	59	0 - 100	••••••••		
Beryllium	< dl	0 - .5			
Bismuth	.2	0 - 30	•		
Cadmium	1.1	0 - 2	••••••••		
Lead	22	0 - 15	•••••••••••••••••		
Mercury	93	0 - 3	••		
Nickel	1.9	0 - 12	••		
Platinum	< dl	0 - 2			
Thallium	.2	0 - 14	•		
Thorium	< dl	0 - 12			
Tin	2.6	0 - 6	••••••		
Tungsten	< dl	0 - 23			
Uranium	< dl	0 - 1			

OTHER TESTS

	Result (mg/dl)	Reference Range (mg/dl)	2 SD Low	1 SD Low	MEAN	1 SD High	2 SD High
Creatinine	42.9	75 - 200	••••••	••••••••	••••••••	••	

Methodology: Analyzed by Induction Coupled Plasma Mass Spectrometry (ICP-MS). Creatinine by Jaffe method.

"dl"=detection limit.
*No safe levels established.

Comments:
(Post provocative challenge.)

Figure 5.3

URINE TOXIC METALS

10/00

LAB#:	CLIENT#:
PATIENT:	DOCTOR: John C. Cline, MD
SEX: Male	Cline Medical Center
AGE: 48	203-1808 Bowen Road
	Nanaimo, BC V9S 5W4 CANADA

POTENTIALLY TOXIC METALS

METALS	RESULT µg/g CREAT	REFERENCE RANGE	WITHIN REFERENCE RANGE	ELEVATED	VERY ELEVATED
Aluminum	< dl	< 35			
Antimony	0.3	< 5	▪		
Arsenic	54	< 100	▬▬▬		
Beryllium	< dl	< 0.5			
Bismuth	0.1	< 30	▪		
Cadmium	< dl	< 2			
Lead	8.5	< 15	▬▬▬▬		
Mercury	19	< 3	▬▬▬▬▬▬▬▬▬▬▬▬▬▬▬▬▬		
Nickel	2.6	< 12	▬▬		
Platinum	< dl	< 2			
Thallium	0.4	< 14			
Thorium	< dl	< 12			
Tin	3.2	< 6			
Tungsten	< dl	< 23			
Uranium	< dl	< 1			

CREATININE

	RESULT mg/dL	REFERENCE RANGE	2SD LOW	1SD LOW	MEAN	1SD HIGH	2SD HIGH
Creatinine	85	75- 200		▬▬▬▬▬▬▬			

SPECIMEN DATA

Comments:

Date Collected:	2/26/2002	Method: ICP-MS		Collection Period:	random
Date Received:	2/28/2002	<dl: less than detection limit		Volume:	
Date Completed:	3/1/2002	Provoking Agent: DMPS		Provocation:	POST PROVOCATIVE

Toxic metals are reported as µg/g creatinine to account for urine dilution variations. **Reference ranges are representative of a healthy population under non-challenge or non-provoked conditions.** No safe reference levels for toxic metals have been established.

©2000 DOCTOR'S DATA, INC. • ADDRESS: 3755 Illinois Avenue, St. Charles, IL 60174-2420 • LABORATORY DIRECTOR: James T. Hicks, MD, Ph.D., FCAP
TOLL FREE: 800.323.2784 • TEL: 630.377.8139 • FAX: 630.587.7860 • EMAIL: inquiries@doctorsdata.com • WEBSITE: www.doctorsdata.com
CLIA ID NO: 14D0646470 • MEDICARE PROVIDER NO: 148453 • TAX ID NO. (FEIN): 93-0941625

Figure 5.4

improvement in his gastrointestinal symptoms, and he felt better in general. At this point, I placed him on large dosages of an excellent probiotic (the friendly bacteria, such as lactobacillus or bifidobacter). We then continued monthly intravenous DMPS injections and added far infrared sauna treatments immediately following the DMPS. At treatment number six, another challenge test was done. It showed a marked increase in the amount of mercury, with the level now being 93 mcg. (see Figure 5.3) This high level indicated that mercury was being flushed out of his system, and so we continued with monthly DMPS treatments. Gradually, Daniel's health improved to the point where he was able to teach full time and perform strenuous sailing with no ill aftereffects. At treatment number eleven, another DMPS challenge test was done, showing a mercury level of 39.

Daniel continued with monthly intravenous DMPS injections and far infrared sauna treatments. At treatment number seventeen, another challenge test showed a marked lowering of mercury to 19 mcg, with negligible amounts of other metals. (see Figure 5.4)

Case Discussion

Daniel's several traumas and surgical procedures produced scar tissue, which in turn produced electric fields in his body. His mercury amalgams and the chemical and metal exposures that he experienced as a heavy-duty diesel mechanic resulted in toxic overload. A further key event was the dysentery he experienced in the Moroccan jail, which set him up for years of disordered gastrointestinal function. The tipping point occurred when he had all his mercury amalgams removed in one sitting at thirty-eight years old. His health tilted negatively and rapidly at that point, and the steps I have described were necessary for him to recover. It was important initially to recognize Daniel's disordered gastrointestinal function and to address this issue with antiparasitic medication and with high-dose probiotics. Removal of toxic metals and chemicals then restored Daniel's system to the positive range. (see Figure 5.5) He presently finds that if he is not careful about what he eats

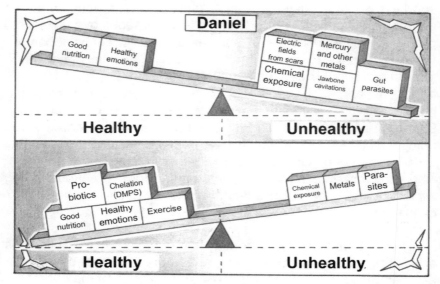

Figure 5.5 Daniel

and neglects to take his probiotics, he can begin to tilt again into the unhealthy state.

Detoxification Organs

Now that I have described the general workings of the gastrointestinal system, I will briefly cover the specific organs that allow us to rid ourselves of toxins – the liver, lungs, kidneys, and skin.

Liver

The liver is the largest internal organ in the body. It is also the only internal organ that can regenerate itself, which gives us a clue to how vital it is. Raw materials come into the liver from the intestine and are funneled into various divisions where many different substances are synthesized, such as lipoproteins, plasma

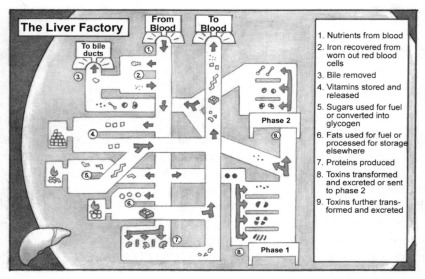

Figure 5.5 The Liver Factory

proteins, clotting factors, glucose, and a storage form of glucose called glycogen. As well, toxins are transformed by the liver so that they are more water soluble and hence more easily excreted.

Converting substances from toxic to nontoxic is carried out by way of a series of chemical reactions in the cells of the liver. These reactions are divided into two phases. In phase one, the chemical reactions remove electrons (oxidation), add electrons (reduction) to toxins, or split toxins into fragments by the addition of water (hydrolysis). These reactions are performed by groups of enzymes known as the cytochrome P450 system. There are likely hundreds of different pathways in this system, and a diverse range of substances, such as petrochemicals, medications, steroid hormones, and the intermediate products of chemical reactions are funneled through these enzymatic pathways. When toxic substances go through these pathways, they are altered and in some cases are ready for direct excretion into the bile. In other cases, they require further transformation and are shunted into phase two detoxification pathways.

There are many phase two detoxification pathways, but they all involve the addition of various molecules to the toxic intermediate substance. This addition of molecules is called conjugation, and each pathway is named after the type of molecule added to the toxic intermediate. For example, if a small protein called glutathione is added, this is the glutathione pathway. If sulfur groups are added, we have the sulfation pathway. If methyl groups are added, we have the methylation pathway, and so on. As it happens, mercury preferentially goes through the glutathione pathway, but two molecules of glutathione are required to bind one ion of mercury. Therefore, if a person is toxic with mercury, the glutathione pathways become depleted very quickly. In general, once the toxic intermediates go through the phase two pathways, they are far less toxic and more water soluble than the original toxic compound, and they are ready for excretion through the bile and into the bowel, or through the blood to the kidneys and into the urine.

It is important to note that if the phase two pathways are disabled in any way, the toxic intermediates coming from the phase one pathways can back up and are then released into the general system. These toxic intermediates are often much more toxic than the original compound, and if they are released into the body, they can have a serious impact on cellular function. Energy production, nervous system function, and immune system function can be adversely affected.

If the multitude of phase one and phase two pathways are to function properly, they must be supplied with the proper nutrients. For example, all enzymes are formed from amino acids, which are the building blocks of proteins. If the diet is low in protein, enzymatic pathways will not function due to a lack of amino acids. Furthermore, if enzymes are inhibited by toxic heavy metals, their action will be blocked, and detoxification will be slowed or even halted.

The phase one and phase two divisions must also be in balance if they are to work efficiently. (see Figure 5.6) If phase one pathways are working too quickly, then the phase two pathways can become overwhelmed by the release of toxic intermediates. For example, substances such as alcohol, tobacco, and certain medications can cause phase one pathways to be overactive. Conversely, medications such as oral birth control pills,

Phase 1 / Phase 2 – Detoxification Scenarios

1	Phase 1 (Normal)	Phase 2 (Normal) = ⇨ Toxins eliminated in bile and urine
2	Phase 1 ⇩	Phase 2 (Normal) = ⇪ Toxic Intermediates into the Body
3	Phase 1 ⇧	Phase 2 (Normal) = ⇪ Toxic Intermediates into the Body
4	Phase 1 (Normal)	Phase 2 ⇩ = ⇪ Toxic Intermediates into the Body

Figure 5.6

antidepressants, and acid production blockers for the stomach can inhibit phase one pathways. Furthermore, if phase one pathways are working normally and phase two pathways are inhibited, a buildup of toxic intermediates can occur. Tests are available to give information about how these pathways are working, and I have found these tests to be invaluable when I am faced with challenging cases.[2]

Another important topic to consider in this context is genetic diversity, which means that we all have slightly different phase one and phase two pathways. Consequently, we differ in our ability to produce the enzymes required in these pathways, a fact which partly accounts for the tremendous variability that is seen in the population when it comes to tolerating medications. For example, a subset of the population is known as slow detoxifiers. These people, when given drug X in the usual dosage, will maintain excessively high levels of the drug within their bodies and will often develop serious and sometimes fatal side effects. Other individuals who have detoxification pathways that work in overdrive are known as fast detoxifiers. When given the usual dosage of drug X, they retain only low levels in their bodies and will not obtain the therapeutic benefit. However, we now have genetic tests enabling us to predict accurately how well a person will be able to detoxify a substance. By using such tests, we should be able to reduce the incidence of adverse effects caused by medication.[3]

Lungs, Kidneys, and Skin

Basically, the lungs allow a close interface between the air we breathe and our cardiovascular system. The air goes down the bronchial tubes into progressively smaller branches until it ends up in tiny air sacs called alveoli. Here a gas exchange takes place, with oxygen going into the system and carbon dioxide (a waste product) coming out. If this exchange does not occur efficiently, a profound impact will rapidly be felt throughout the body. Breathing properly is not only life sustaining, but it is also fundamentally important for detoxification.

Likewise, our kidneys constantly filter and clean our blood, eliminating many toxic substances from both external and internal sources. One of the most important things we can do to improve kidney function is to drink an adequate amount of pure water each day. Some estimates indicate that we should drink half of our body weight in ounces of water each day. Thus, a 160-pound person would require eighty ounces of water per day, which works out to ten eight-ounce glasses of water.[4]

Another important principle is to avoid consuming things that can have an adverse effect on kidney function. For example, anti-inflammatory medications (NonSteroidal Anti-Inflammatory Drugs, or NSAIDs) are often used in the relief of arthritic symptoms. These can be prescribed by a physician or purchased over the counter. Long-term use of this type of medication can damage the kidneys and result in decreased detoxification ability, increased blood pressure, and even kidney failure.

The skin is the body's largest organ, and one of its main functions is to protect us from the external environment. Yet the skin also detoxifies by excreting toxins such as heavy metals and organic pollutants. Many cultures around the world value therapies that result in increased sweating, and most of us are familiar with saunas, of which there are several types. At our clinic we have a far infrared sauna that has been an important tool in helping our patients detoxify. In this type of sauna, high temperatures are not required in order to obtain the full therapeutic benefit. Many of our patients with chronic fatigue syndrome and fibromyalgia cannot tolerate high temperatures, but in a far infrared sauna, profuse sweating occurs and intracellular toxins are released so that the skin becomes like a "third kidney." Many patients are so impressed by how good they feel after using the far infrared sauna that they purchase their own units to use at home.

Finally, let us not forget how important regular exercise is as a detoxification strategy. Most patients who come to our clinic are feeling so sick and tired that exercise is not a priority. We have observed that once they begin to detoxify, they naturally begin to increase their physical activity. We were designed to be physically active, and regular exercise enhances cellular detoxification as well as the function of all the detoxification organs.[5]

Summary

It is important to have a broad idea of how our bodies perform the vital function of detoxification so that we can take steps to improve the health and integrity of our gastrointestinal system. This might require detecting and eliminating foods that are causing inflammation and restoring the integrity of the lining of the intestine by the addition of nutritious foods, nutritional supplements, and probiotic bacteria. A toxic load will then be taken off the liver, which can be further supported through diet and by the addition of certain key nutrients found in medical food products. The lungs, kidneys, and skin are also important detoxification organs, and we should care for them well. To conclude this chapter and to highlight the basic importance of our gastrointestinal health, let me tell you about a woman whom we will call Jillian.

Jillian's Case

When I first met her, Jillian was in her early sixties. Although her marriage was happy, she had experienced years of stress from poor relationships with her extended family. For decades, she had problems with chronic daily headaches that sometimes deteriorated into migraines. She would often burp and get bloated after consuming food. Her bowel function was irregular, and she often had excessive gas. Her energy was poor, and she required several naps during the day. Her mood was often depressed, and she experienced pain in her muscles and joints. Over the course of several decades, she had gained significant weight. Also, all her teeth had been removed, and she now wore dentures. She had always worked from home, and it was evident that she had not been exposed to any unusual sources of toxins. She had traveled in Southeast Asia but did not develop any illnesses during her travels.

Jillian's family physician told her that she was depressed and placed her on a series of antidepressant medications, which she was unable to tolerate and which resulted in further weight gain. On examining her, I concluded that she appeared tired rather than depressed, and, other than the fact that she was obese, her examination and standard laboratory tests (blood, urine, and stool) were unremarkable.

I decided initially to treat Jillian with an elimination diet together with a medical food called <u>RevitalX ®,</u> which is designed to rejuvenate the lining of the intestine. Within one week she began to feel better, and she noticed that she was not experiencing headaches. By the end of the second week, she had no more gastrointestinal symptoms, her muscle and joint pains resolved, her energy increased, and she was no longer napping during the day. She reported also that she was able to do various jobs around her house and yard. Interestingly, during the fourth week she cheated on her diet and consumed wheat and dairy products. Within one day, most of her symptoms returned, especially the headaches and low energy. Fortunately, she recognized the connection between consumption of certain foods and her symptom complex.

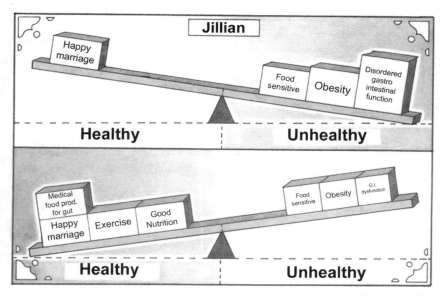

Figure 5.7 Jillian

It was quite clear to me that for many decades Jillian had been consuming foods that were resulting in chronic inflammation in the lining of her intestine, resulting in a "leaky gut." The increased toxic load on her liver, followed by the release of toxins into her system, caused the symptoms I have described above.

---

[1] Jaffe R, Mani J, DeVane J, Mani H. Tolerance loss in diabetics: association with foreign antigen exposure. Diabet Med. 2006 Aug; 23(8):924-5. www.elisaact.com

[2] More information about detoxification profile testing available at www.genovadx.com.

[3] For more information on this topic, go to www.genovations.com.

[4] Batmanghelidj, F. Your Body's Many Cries for Water. Global Health Solutions, Inc. 2003.

[5] Astrofit. Evans, W., Couzens, GS: Free Press, a division of Simon and Shuster; 2002.

The Many Faces of Mercury

Widespread low-level mercury exposure in the general population has increased markedly in recent years because of three specific sources: dental mercury amalgams (silver fillings), which are the most common source of exposure; ethyl mercury (thimerosal) in vaccines; and dietary intake of mercury-contaminated fish. Also, the environment in general has become increasingly contaminated as a result of mercury released from coal-burning electric power plants, mining, pulp and paper industries, and incineration of municipal, medical, and dental waste.[1]

Ignorance about the extreme danger of mercury has contributed significantly to the problem of widespread contamination. We have seen something of this ignorance in the distressing example of the HMS Triumph, which I discussed in Chapter 3. A further, not dissimilar example is the contamination of lighthouses by toxic fumes given off by the mercury bath in which the large light was suspended. Outside the lighthouses, storage barrels were filled with liquid mercury that lighthouse keepers would carry up to the light in order to replenish the mercury that was constantly vaporizing. We hear of lighthouse keepers going mad because of isolation, but I suspect that they were suffering from mercury toxicity.

The sailors on the Triumph and the keepers of remote lighthouses might seem far removed from our own day-to-day experience, and yet it is highly probable that most of us have been directly exposed to mercury. The majority of my patients tell me that they remember playing with liquid mercury obtained from a broken thermometer, and I expect the same holds true for many readers of this book. Additionally, a large percentage of the population is exposed to mercury through dental amalgams. For the most part, people do not think very much about the consequences of such exposure, even though it has been well established since the 1980s that mercury vapor is continuously released from amalgam fillings. According to the World Health Organization, the daily human exposure to mercury vapor from amalgam fillings ranges from 3 to 17 micrograms, compared to a maximum of 2.6 micrograms from all other sources.[2] Patrick Stortebecker, MD, PhD, pointedly asks whether or not "the majority of the population in Western industrialized countries suffers from a slowly developing mercury poisoning," and he concludes that, with all probability, the "answer is yes!"[3]

Typical symptoms of mercury poisoning are extreme fatigue (both physical and mental), increased irritability, moodiness marked by unpredictable and sudden outbursts of anger, lack of concentration, self-effacement combined with lack of self-confidence, loss of initiative, timidity, shyness, introversion, unmotivated anxiety, and depression. Who among Westerners, we might ask, is not suffering, more or less, from some symptoms of these abnormalities so highly typical of chronic mercury intoxication?

Clear scientific evidence indicates that the limits for the values of maximum allowable concentrations of mercury are often far surpassed, mainly due to mercury released from dental amalgams. Dental mercury amalgams are not stable, although it is often claimed that they are; rather, they undergo corrosion, and dangerous amounts of mercury vapor are released daily, especially when we chew. Moreover, it has been established that high concentrations of metallic mercury found postmortem in the brain originate mainly from the mercury harbored in our dental amalgam fillings. These fillings release vapor that may be inhaled and in that way enter the general blood circulation and pass into the body.

Even more dangerous are mercury fumes that settle on the mucous membranes of the upper region of the nasal cavity. From there the mercury is transported directly to the brain through the olfactory nerves (the cranial nerves that provide us with a sense of smell) or through the valveless cranial venous system that presents an open communication between the oral and nasal cavity and the brain. Another important route lies through the trigeminal nerves running from the teeth directly to the brain stem.

Mercury Species

Mercury exists in various forms, or species. The first is elemental. This is the familiar shiny, slithery beads of liquid that most of us know from playing with a broken thermometer. The second is organic and is formed when mercury is joined to various carbon atoms to produce methyl mercury, dimethyl mercury, ethyl mercury, and so on. The third is inorganic, and this is formed when mercury is joined to inorganic substances such as iodide, sulfide, chloride, and oxide. The body handles these different forms of mercury in different ways, as is illustrated in Figure 6.1 below.

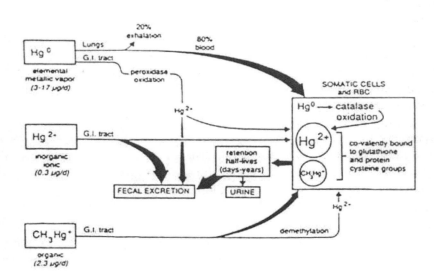

Figure 6.1 Metabolism of Mercury Species[1]

Elemental Mercury

Elemental mercury vaporizes rapidly from liquid mercury at room temperature and is readily inhaled. Eighty percent of the vapor goes directly to the bloodstream, which transports it throughout the body. A smaller percentage goes to the brain through the nerves in the superior part of our nostrils. This form of mercury is called lipophilic, which means "fat loving," and it easily crosses cell membranes and pervades lipid rich tissues such as the nervous system, the glands, the liver, and the kidneys. Lipophilic mercury is one of the most toxic forms of mercury, and the historical case about the British sailors that I reviewed in Chapter 3 is an example of how dangerous it is. A more modern example is a recently published study showing that in children there is a clear-cut relationship between body burdens of mercury and acute eczema. That is, children with amalgam fillings were found to exhibit significantly higher urinary mercury concentrations than children without amalgams. The higher the urinary mercury concentration, the higher the risk for acute eczematous lesions.[4]

Organic Mercury

Methylmercury comes primarily from the ingestion of contaminated fish. Inorganic mercury from the seabed is converted into methylmercury by microorganisms such as bacteria, phytoplankton, and fungi. As fish eat these organisms, the methylmercury rises up the food chain, becoming concentrated in the larger and older saltwater fish such as swordfish, shark, tuna (although the smaller ones such as albacore are generally safe), and halibut (again, smaller ones less than fifty pounds are generally safe), and in freshwater fish such as pike, walleye, and bass.[5] A basic principle to remember is this: the older and larger the fish, the more mercury tends to accumulate in its tissues. Consumption of fish containing mercury results in a 95 percent absorption of methylmercury across the gastrointestinal tract. This form of mercury is also lipophilic and concentrates in the nervous system.

If pregnant women consume fish containing mercury, the developing nervous system of the fetus will be adversely affected. In the last few years repeated warnings issued by regulatory agencies have advised women to avoid consumption of certain fish (as listed above) during pregnancy. In March 2004, the FDA-EPA released a consumer advisory targeted at pregnant women, women who may become pregnant, nursing mothers, and young children. These groups are advised to avoid consumption of shark, swordfish, king mackerel, and tilefish. Recent studies on children from the Faroe Islands show measurable adverse health effects, such as heart rhythm disturbances and abnormal neurological function. The reason seems to be that their mothers consumed mercury-contaminated fish during pregnancy.[6] A quick source of accurate information on the mercury content of various types of fish can be viewed at www.gotmercury.org.

One of the most famous incidents of acute mercury toxicity from fish ingestion occurred at Minimata Bay in Japan during the 1950s. The fish in this area became contaminated with commercial effluent containing mercury. Many people living on the bay ate the fish and also became contaminated. One hundred and twenty of these people developed severe brain damage, and 1,422 infants who appeared healthy at birth were later found to have profound neurological problems. Thousands of follow-up cases resulting from this catastrophe have been identified, and a clinical syndrome, Minimata disease, has been named after the incident.

Ethyl Mercury

Another form of organic mercury that has raised a great deal of concern and controversy is ethyl mercury, also known as thimerisol. Since the 1930s, thimerisol has been a preservative of choice in the manufacture of vaccines, and there is now compelling evidence linking the use of vaccines containing thimerisol with a number of childhood neurological conditions, such as the autistic spectrum of disorders.[7] In 1999 the American Academy of Pediatrics and the

U.S. Public Health Service raised concern about the safety of ethyl mercury used in vaccinations.

Inorganic Mercury

In Chapter 3, I wrote briefly about the main form of inorganic mercury, namely cinnabar ore or mercuric sulfide. When cinnabar is refined, it produces volatile elemental mercury, which is highly toxic. Elemental mercury can also be converted into inorganic mercury compounds that are used in the production of fungicides. It is also used in the production of mercuric iodide, an ingredient used in skin-lightening creams. Mercuric chloride has been used as a topical antiseptic and a disinfecting agent, and it was once an ingredient in medicinal products that included laxatives, deworming medications, and even teething powders. You may remember using mercurochrome on your skin as an antiseptic; if so, you might now be disturbed to learn that it contained 2 percent mercury. Mercuric sulfide and mercuric oxide have also been used as coloring agents in paints, and mercuric sulfide is one of the red coloring agents in tattoo dyes.

In summary, products to watch out for are: tuna (the smaller ones such as albacore are generally safe), swordfish, halibut (under fifty pounds are generally safe), various cosmetics, medications, personal use items, certain hair dyes, mercurochrome, calomel, some powders, talcs, contact lens solutions, latex paints, floor waxes and polishes, wood preservatives, tattoos, various batteries, and fungicides. People employed in certain occupations are also more likely to be exposed to mercury. Examples are instrument technicians, dentists and dental assistants, farmers, fungicide makers, miners, paint makers, pesticide workers, thermometer makers, and lighthouse keepers.

Why Mercury Is So Toxic and How It Affects Us

When mercury enters our cells, it attaches to proteins, which are made from amino acids, and many amino acids contain sulfur groups to which mercury binds. Enzymes are specialized proteins that enable key chemical reactions to go forward, and these enzymes have a specific structure or configuration. By binding to the sulfur groups in the enzymes, mercury irreversibly alters the structure of the enzymes themselves and effectively inhibits their function. Also, nerve cells require a structural protein called tubulin to enable information transfer to occur. But when mercury binds to the enzyme required to produce tubulin, the structure is destroyed, and the information transfer cannot occur.[8] (see Figure 6.2) Because all of our bodily processes require enzymes, the number of chemical reactions that are inhibited is very great.

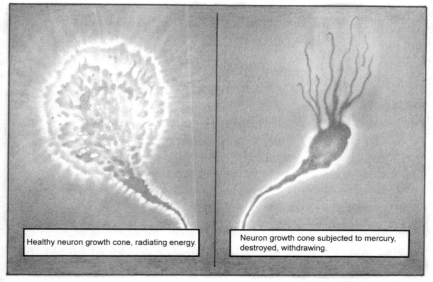

Healthy neuron growth cone, radiating energy.

Neuron growth cone subjected to mercury, destroyed, withdrawing.

Figure 6.2 The Effect of Mercury on Nerves

In turn, because the number of cellular processes that can be disrupted by mercury is also very great, the symptoms that can be caused by mercury toxicity are bewilderingly varied. Over 200 symptoms have been associated with mercury toxicity, which, consequently, has many faces or presentations. As I have mentioned, this is the reason mercury has been called the "great masquerader." Unless a health practitioner is alert to the hazards of mercury when meeting with a patient, the diagnosis is often missed. Heather's case provides a compelling example of the harmful effects of mercury and also how easily misdiagnosis can occur.

Heather's Case

Heather was a thirty-five-year-old hairstylist who read a newspaper article about our work with detoxification. She told me that she had been completely well until she was thirteen years old. At that time, she suddenly developed hives over most of her body. Also, she often experienced swelling of her lips and eyelids. Over the next twenty-two years, she experienced hives on a daily basis, and the winter before I met her, she had taken ten trips to the emergency room for injections of adrenaline and steroids. She had been placed on long-term prednisone five times, which barely controlled her symptoms and resulted in a weight gain of 110 pounds. When her symptom complex began, her platelet count suddenly dropped, but numerous tests failed to disclose any underlying cause.

Heather suffered from daily headaches, as well as from fatigue that gradually became profound. Over time, she developed generalized muscle and joint pains, sleep disturbances, gastrointestinal dysfunction, and chronic flu-like symptoms. When she was twenty-eight years old she was diagnosed with fibromyalgia by a rheumatologist. When we met, Heather's medications included an antihistamine taken eight times per day.

Heather's medical history revealed that she had all of her childhood immunizations. She had a tonsillectomy at two years old, lymph node excision from the left neck at five years old, and left trigger thumb repair and tubal ligation at thirty-three years old. She had been a smoker but gave up cigarettes when she was thirty-four. In her late teens, she consumed a lot of alcohol and used marijuana. When I met her, she was happily married, had one child, and was working as a hairstylist. Her family physician forwarded copies of all investigations, which were within normal limits. Interestingly, her blood mercury level was low (3 nmol/L, with normal being 0-49).

The key question I posed in Heather's case was whether or not she had any dental procedures prior to the onset of her symptoms. Her answer was very revealing, because, as I have noted, she was very healthy until thirteen years of age, but precisely at that time her dentist told her that she would require braces. She was also advised that because she had cavities in her teeth she would require mercury amalgams. Subsequently, over a two-month period, she had twelve mercury amalgams placed during several sessions. She told me that after each session she felt sick for days. The braces were then placed, and shortly thereafter she developed the severe symptom complex described above. One week before coming to my clinic she had several mercury amalgams removed and replaced with composite material, but she reported that after these replacements her fatigue became much worse.

When I examined her, Heather had several small patches of hives on her arms and legs. Her hands were cool to touch. I counted nine mercury amalgams in her mouth, but no crowns or root canals were present. Sixteen out of eighteen fibromyalgia tender points were positive.

Heather's Treatment

I placed Heather on a diet and a nutritional supplementary program. A DMPS Challenge Test showed a very high level of mercury in the urine (210 mcg, with normal being less than 3). Lead was slightly elevated at 17 (normal being less than 15). Tin was elevated at 8.9 (normal being less than 6). (see Figure 6.4) Heather then received a series of monthly intravenous DMPS injections, the first three in conjunction with the careful removal of her amalgams. By her sixth treatment, she reported that she was experiencing hives infrequently, and her energy had increased so significantly that she was working out at a gym several times a week. During a period of six months, she lost twenty-two pounds, and her muscle and joint pain improved considerably.

At treatment number six, a DMPS Challenge Test showed that Heather's urinary mercury level had dropped to 17, lead to 13, and tin to 4.2. By her ninth treatment she announced that she was feeling well and had not experienced hives for several months. Her muscle and joint pains had also resolved completely.

Case Discussion

Heather was well until she was thirteen years old, even though her childhood vaccinations had exposed her to ethyl mercury. But when she turned thirteen, a major toxic exposure occurred with the placement of the twelve mercury amalgams combined with the metallic braces. This mixture of metals in her mouth set up an electric field produced by galvanic forces (more about galvanism in the chapter on electromagnetic fields) and the scars from her surgical procedures would possibly have produced the same effect. Heather's work as a hairstylist exposed her to a range of chemicals present in various hair care products. She was a smoker until she was thirty-four years old, and she had consumed a lot of alcohol and some marijuana before she was eighteen. For a period of some twenty-two years, she had taken a wide variety of medications. Not

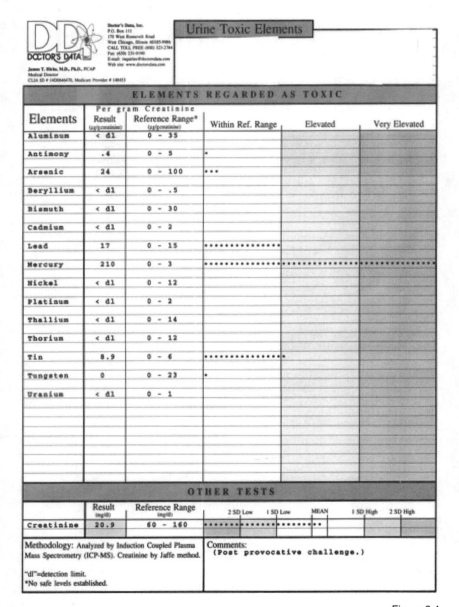

Figure 6.4

surprisingly, the cumulative effect of these various events caused the left side of the balance to tilt downward, Heather's detoxification systems were quickly overwhelmed, and she experienced a rapid deterioration in health.

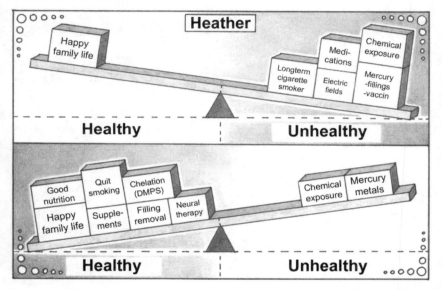

Figure 6.3 Heather

Although mercury played an important role in bringing about Heather's ill health, it was just one among several factors, and its destructive impact could all too easily be overlooked. Here we should recall that the blood mercury reading forwarded by Heather's physician was low. Again, mercury, "the great masquerader," remains elusive; the fact is that blood mercury readings often do not indicate the extent of actual contamination. This is because mercury moves rapidly from the blood, concentrating instead within our cells and lipid-rich tissues.

Because mercury toxicity is such an important subject, another case presentation is warranted, so let me introduce you to Simon.

Simon's Case

Simon was a thirty-nine-year-old saw operator who had worked for the previous fourteen years at an aluminum smelter and was also a part-time fishing guide. He presented with one of the worst cases of eczema I have ever seen. He told me that since early childhood he had continuous problems with eczema affecting his forehead, scalp, neck, elbows, forearms, hands, back, and lower legs. Over time, he also developed hives on his skin. As a child, he was given almonds, and within minutes he fainted and his throat swelled shut. From that time, he meticulously avoided eating almonds as well as hazelnuts, to which he was also highly sensitive. For the six years before I met him, Simon's symptoms became gradually worse, and during the preceding three months they had become unbearable. In order to control his symptoms, he had to take Benadryl (an oral antihistamine) several times each day and apply potent steroid creams and ointments. In the springtime, he developed symptoms of allergic rhinitis when exposed to tree and grass pollens, and the consumption of certain foods such as eggs and salmon made his skin condition worse. He mentioned that when exposed to cat dander he would start to wheeze.

Over the years, Simon had been prescribed many different types of antihistamines, topical steroid creams, and antibiotics. He visited several allergists, whose tests revealed severe reactions to trees and grasses. He had moderate reactions also to dust, cat and dog dander, and molds. Skin testing revealed adverse reactions to cashews, almonds, hazelnuts, sesame, dairy, wheat, and shellfish. Blood tests revealed very high levels of Immunoglobulin E (IgE) (9540 microgram/L, with normal being 0-430), indicating that his immune system was very reactive and in a hyperalert state.

Simon consulted internal medicine specialists in the U.S. and Canada, but no matter which specialist he saw, the diagnosis was the same: severe atopic dermatitis, urticaria (hives), angioedema (severe hives with local tissue swelling), and allergic rhinitis. When

I first met him, he was desperate to find an effective treatment because the severity of his condition was having a major impact on his life. He had chronic sleep disturbances because of severe itching, his energy fluctuated, and he had difficulty maintaining his weight. Nevertheless, despite all these problems, he enjoyed playing hockey and tennis, as well as lifting weights.

Simon's past history revealed that his mother had mercury amalgams present in her mouth when she was pregnant with him. He had gotten all his childhood vaccinations, and he began getting mercury amalgams placed in his teeth as a child. He therefore would have accumulated some mercury from his mother, from the vaccines, and especially from the eleven amalgams present in his teeth. He had also consumed plentiful amounts of fish, from which, again, he would have absorbed mercury. He had worked at the aluminum smelter for fourteen years, and for the first seven years his job involved pouring liquid aluminum alloy that exposed him to fumes containing metals.

When I examined him, Simon had severe eczema on his forehead, scalp, neck, elbows, forearms, hands, and lower legs, but his examination was otherwise unremarkable. We performed skin testing for inhalants and found that he had severe reactions to dust mites, cat, dog, guinea pig, and horse danders, as well as to cockroaches. He also exhibited severe reactions to trees, grasses, and weeds, and he had moderate reactions to molds. I ordered a number of investigations which showed that his IgE level was still critically elevated (3908 microgram/L, with normal being 0-430). Stool testing was negative for parasites, and his laboratory work was otherwise unremarkable.

Simon was placed on the dietary protocol I have described earlier, together with nutritional supplements. His first DMPS challenge test showed a mercury level of 320 mcg (with normal being less than 3). Aluminum was elevated (44, with normal being less than 35). Lead was elevated (15, with normal being less than

URINE TOXIC METALS

10/00

POTENTIALLY TOXIC METALS

TOXIC METALS	RESULT µg/g CREAT	REFERENCE RANGE	WITHIN REFERENCE RANGE	ELEVATED	VERY ELEVATED
Aluminum	44	< 35			
Antimony	< dl	< 5			
Arsenic	60	< 100			
Beryllium	< dl	< 0.5			
Bismuth	< dl	< 30			
Cadmium	2.1	< 2			
Lead	15	< 15			
Mercury	320	< 3			
Nickel	6.4	< 12			
Platinum	< dl	< 2			
Thallium	0.6	< 14			
Thorium	< dl	< 12			
Tin	2.7	< 6			
Tungsten	0.8	< 23			
Uranium	< dl	< 1			

CREATININE

	RESULT mg/dL	REFERENCE RANGE	2SD LOW	1SD LOW	MEAN	1SD HIGH	2SD HIGH
Creatinine	13	75 - 200					

SPECIMEN DATA

Comments:

Date Collected:	9/21/2001	Method:	ICP-MS	Collection Period:	random
Date Received:	9/25/2001	<dl:	less than detection limit	Volume:	
Date Completed:	9/28/2001			Provocation:	POST PROVOCATIVE

Toxic metals are reported as µg/g creatinine to account for urine dilution variations. Reference ranges are representative of a healthy population under non-challenge or non-provoked conditions. No safe reference levels for toxic metals have been established.

©2000 DOCTOR'S DATA, INC. • ADDRESS: 3755 Illinois Avenue, St. Charles, IL 60174-2420 • LABORATORY DIRECTOR: James T. Hicks, MD, Ph.D., FCAP
TOLL FREE: 800.323.2784 • TEL: 630.377.8139 • FAX: 630.587.7860 • EMAIL: inquiries@doctorsdata.com • WEBSITE: www.doctorsdata.com
CLIA ID NO: 14D0646470 • MEDICARE PROVIDER NO: 148453 • TAX ID NO. (FEIN): 93-0941625

Figure 6.5

DETOXIFY FOR LIFE

URINE TOXIC METALS

POTENTIALLY TOXIC METALS

METALS	RESULT µg/g CREAT	REFERENCE RANGE	WITHIN REFERENCE RANGE	ELEVATED	VERY ELEVATED
Aluminum	12	< 35			
Antimony	< dl	< 5			
Arsenic	41	< 100			
Beryllium	< dl	< 0.5			
Bismuth	9.4	< 30			
Cadmium	0.4	< 2			
Lead	2.8	< 15			
Mercury	81	< 3			
Nickel	1.3	< 12			
Platinum	< dl	< 2			
Thallium	0.4	< 14			
Thorium	< dl	< 12			
Tin	0.4	< 6			
Tungsten	0.1	< 23			
Uranium	< dl	< 1			

CREATININE

	RESULT mg/dL	REFERENCE RANGE	2SD LOW	1SD LOW	MEAN	1SD HIGH	2SD HIGH
Creatinine	79	75- 200					

SPECIMEN DATA

Comments:
Date Collected:	4/9/2002	Method:	ICP-MS	Collection Period:	random
Date Received:	4/11/2002	<dl:	less than detection limit	Volume:	
Date Completed:	4/17/2002	Provoking Agent:	DMPS	Provocation:	POST PROVOCATIVE

Toxic metals are reported as µg/g creatinine to account for urine dilution variations. **Reference ranges are representative of a healthy population under non-challenge or non-provoked conditions.** No safe reference levels for toxic metals have been established.

V10.00

©2000-02 DOCTOR'S DATA, INC. • ADDRESS: 3755 Illinois Avenue, St. Charles, IL 60174-2420 • CLIA ID NO: 14D0646470 • MEDICARE PROVIDER NO: 148453
TOLL FREE: 800.323.2784 • TEL: 630.377.8139 • FAX: 630.587.7860 • EMAIL: inquiries@doctorsdata.com • WEBSITE: www.doctorsdata.com

Figure 6.6

5). Cadmium was also elevated (2.1, with normal being less than 2.0). Arsenic, cadmium, nickel, and tin also showed up in his urine, all within the reference range with the exception of cadmium, which was just over the borderline. (see Figure 6.5)

Simon agreed to go ahead with a mercury and heavy metal detoxification program, which initially involved attending a biological dentist on a monthly basis for careful removal of mercury from his teeth. In conjunction with each dental treatment, he came to my clinic for an intravenous injection of DMPS, which circulated through his system at the same time as he was getting his amalgams removed.

After the first few treatments of DMPS combined with dental work, Simon's eczema flared up for approximately two weeks. After his fourth treatment, his skin appeared healthier, and there was much less eczema present. Simon continued to have flare-ups after his dental work and DMPS treatments, but his skin continued to improve. On his seventh treatment, a DMPS challenge revealed a marked drop in the amounts of metals excreted. Mercury was 81, aluminum was 12, and lead was 2.8. Other metals were extremely low. (see Figure 6.6)

Because Simon was improving steadily, we decided to continue with his detoxification program, and after his ninth treatment he reported that he was no longer experiencing symptoms of allergic rhinitis and could expose himself to cat and dog dander without reacting. He was also able to eat salmon and eggs without adverse effects. His weight was increasing, and he noticed no asthma symptoms while playing hockey. His eczema continued to improve, and he stated that his skin condition was now the best it had ever been.

At treatment number ten, Simon showed such improvement that we added far infrared sauna, which he tolerated well. His eczema was now completely absent, and he was able to eat most

URINE TOXIC METALS

POTENTIALLY TOXIC METALS

METALS	RESULT µg/g CREAT	REFERENCE RANGE	WITHIN REFERENCE RANGE	ELEVATED	VERY ELEVATED
Aluminum	< dl	< 35			
Antimony	0.2	< 5	▮		
Arsenic	62	< 100	▬▬▬▬▬		
Beryllium	< dl	< 0.5			
Bismuth	0.1	< 30	▸		
Cadmium	0.2	< 2	▬		
Lead	4.3	< 15	▬▬		
Mercury	82	< 3	▬▬▬▬▬▬▬▬▬▬▬▬▬▬▬		
Nickel	2.9	< 12	▬▬		
Platinum	< dl	< 2			
Thallium	0.4	< 14	▮		
Thorium	< dl	< 12			
Tin	0.9	< 6	▬		
Tungsten	0.2	< 23	▸		
Uranium	0.03	< 1	▮		

CREATININE

	RESULT mg/dL	REFERENCE RANGE	2SD LOW	1SD LOW	MEAN	1SD HIGH	2SD HIGH
Creatinine	150	75- 200			▬▬		

SPECIMEN DATA

Comments:

Date Collected:	7/4/2003	Method:	ICP-MS	Collection Period:	Random
Date Received:	7/9/2003	<dl:	less than detection limit	Volume:	1035 ml
Date Completed:	7/11/2003	Provoking Agent:	DMPS	Provocation:	POST PROVOCATIVE

Toxic metals are reported as µg/g creatinine to account for urine dilution variations. **Reference ranges are representative of a healthy population under non-challenge or non-provoked conditions.** No safe reference levels for toxic metals have been established.

V10.00

©DOCTOR'S DATA, INC. • ADDRESS: 3755 Illinois Avenue, St. Charles, IL 60174-2420 • CLIA ID NO: 14D0646470 • MEDICARE PROVIDER NO: 148453

Figure 6.7

URINE TOXIC METALS

POTENTIALLY TOXIC METALS

METALS	RESULT µg/g CREAT	REFERENCE RANGE	WITHIN REFERENCE RANGE	ELEVATED	VERY ELEVATED
Aluminum	< dl	< 25			
Antimony	0.2	< 0.6			
Arsenic	19	< 120			
Beryllium	< dl	< 0.5			
Bismuth	< dl	< 10			
Cadmium	0.3	< 2			
Lead	2.8	< 5			
Mercury	3.9	< 3			
Nickel	1.5	< 10			
Platinum	< dl	< 1			
Thallium	0.2	< 0.7			
Thorium	< dl	< 0.3			
Tin	0.9	< 9			
Tungsten	0.02	< 0.7			
Uranium	< dl	< 0.1			

CREATININE

	RESULT mg/dL	REFERENCE RANGE	2SD LOW 1SD LOW	MEAN	1SD HIGH 2SD HIGH
Creatinine	160	45- 225			

SPECIMEN DATA

Comments:

Date Collected:	6/21/2005	Method: ICP-MS		Collection Period:	Random
Date Received:	6/22/2005	<dl: less than detection limit		Volume:	1220 ml
Date Completed:	6/24/2005	Provoking Agent: DMPS		Provocation:	POST PROVOCATIVE

Toxic metals are reported as µg/g creatinine to account for urine dilution variations. **Reference ranges are representative of a healthy population under non-challenge or non-provoked conditions.** No safe reference levels for toxic metals have been established. V10.00

Figure 6.8

foods to which he had previously reacted. I told him that he should learn to rotate these foods on a four-day cycle to help prevent the allergies from returning. I also mentioned that he should continue to avoid consumption of nuts because he had severe life-threatening reactions to them.

On treatment number twelve, the DMPS challenge test showed that Simon's mercury level was still high (82), but levels of the other metals were low. (see Figure 6.7) I interpreted these findings to mean that he was still excreting significant amounts of mercury, and I suggested to Simon that he might consider purchasing a far infrared sauna for his own use. He did so, and subsequently used the sauna two or three times per week. I also placed him on an excellent oral heavy-metal chelating agent called penicillamine, which he took in small dosages two days per week for a two-month period. We performed his final DMPS challenge test, and his mercury level had fallen to 3.9, lead was 2.8, and he had negligible levels of all other metals. (see Figure 6.8)

During the previous spring, Simon had experienced only mild symptoms of allergic rhinitis. He was now in the midst of a busy fishing season, and found that when he handled a lot of fish he developed mild eczema on his hands. He was able to tolerate most foods and was consuming organic plain yogurt daily as well as eight eggs per week. He was sleeping well, was very active in sports, and generally happy with life. Over the long-term, I advised him to eat well, get sufficient sleep, remain physically active, avoid mercury as much as possible, and continue with far infrared sauna treatments on a regular basis.

Case Discussion

Simon's case demonstrates how reactive the immune system can become with exposure to various toxins. Once again, using the TILT Phenomenon model we see that as Simon progressed through life, his exposure to, and accumulation of toxins gradually increased. He was already exposed to mercury in his mother's womb, as well as by way of his childhood vaccinations. Visits to the dentist during childhood further increased the mercury in his system, and his balance began to tilt to the left. Working at the aluminum smelter increased his toxic load significantly, so much so that Simon's allergic reactions progressed to the point where he began a desperate search for answers. Only after the removal of a significant amount of toxins, and especially mercury, was his system able to tilt back into the healthy zone.

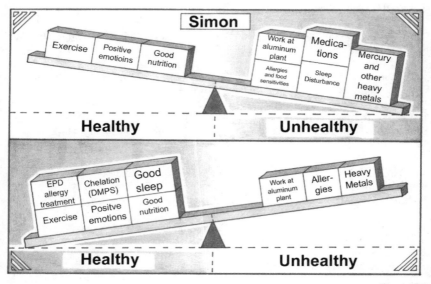

Figure 6.9

[1] Lorscheider, F.L., Vimy, M.J., Summers, A.O. Mercury exposure from silver tooth fillings: emerging evidence questions a traditional dental paradigm. FASEB Journal 1995; 9:504-508.

Geier DA, Geier MR. A comparative evaluation of the effects of MMR immunization and mercury doses from thimerosal-containing childhood vaccines on the population prevalence of autism. Med Sci Monit. 2004 Mar 1; 10(3).

Clarkson, T.W., The three faces of mercury, Environ Health Perspect. 2002; 110 (supplement 1): 11-23.

Krantz A, Dorevitch S. Metal exposure and common chronic diseases: a guide for the clinician. Dis Mon. 2004 May; 50(5): 220-62.

[2] World Health Organization (1992) Environmental Health Criteria 118, Inorganic Mercury (Friberg L., ed), WHO, Geneva.

[3] Stortebecker P. 1985. Mercury Poisoning from Dental Amalgam – a Hazard to Human Brain. Stortebecker Foundation for Research. Sweden.

[4] Weidinger S, Body burden of mercury is associated with acute atopic eczema and total IgE in children from southern Germany. J Allergy Clin Immunol. 2004 Aug; 114(2): 457-9.

[5] Toxicological Profile For Mercury, U.S. Department of Health and Human Services, Public Health Service, Agency for Toxic Substances and Disease Registry. 1999; 1-676. http://www.atsdr.cdc.gov.

[6] Committee on the Toxicological Effects of Methylmercury. Board on Environmental Studies and Toxicology, Commission on Life Sciences. National Research Council. 2000. Toxicological Effects of Methylmercury. Washington, DC:National Academy Press. Available: http://www.nap.edu/books/0309071402/html/

Grandjean P, et al., Cardiac autonomic activity in methylmercury neurotoxicity: 14-year follow-up of a Faroese birth cohort. J Pediatr. 2004 Feb; 144(2): 169-76.

[7] Geier DA, Geier MR. An assessment of downward trends in neurodevelopmental disorders in the United States following removal of thimerosal from childhood vaccines. Med Sci Monit. 2006 Jun; 12(6):CR231-9.

Geier DA, Geier MR. A case series of children with apparent mercury toxic encephalopathies manifesting with clinical symptoms of regressive autistic disorders. J Toxicol Environ Health A. 2007 May 15; 70(10):837-51.

[8] Leong CC, Syed NI, Lorscheider FL. Retrograde degeneration of neurite membrane structural integrity of nerve growth cones following in vitro exposure to mercury. Neuroreport. 2001 Mar 26; 12(4):733-7.

Get the Lead Out

Lead is a blue-gray, soft, malleable heavy metal with physical and chemical properties that make it useful for a wide variety of industrial applications.[1] Yet lead is also toxic, although its harmful effects have frequently been ignored or imperfectly understood. I have read reports that the ancient Roman elite coated their eating and drinking utensils with lead, and I have spoken with retired European plumbers who have told me about constructing rain gutters and lining them with molten lead. I have interviewed retired pipe fitters and plumbers who have also told me about exposure to vapors from pots of molten lead close beside them in poorly ventilated areas.

Not surprisingly, given the many industrial applications of this useful metal, during the past few hundred years, the levels of lead in the general population have increased significantly. We know this because lead levels in bones of healthy modern day people are 1,000 times higher than levels found in the skeletons of people who lived 500 years ago. There is no safe level of lead for humans, and in 2005 the U.S. Department of Health and Human Services added lead to its list of carcinogens.[2]

Still, it is important also to note that in North America, lead levels in adults and children have begun to decline over the past three decades.[3] This decline is the result of a concerted effort to remove lead from gasoline, interior paints, and food cans.[4] Nevertheless, lead persists in old plumbing and in lead paint, as well as in the soil, and low-level lead exposure continues to be a problem.[5] For example, in 1997, data from the U.S. National Health and Nutrition Examination Surveys showed that 4.4 percent of the children in the

United States had elevated blood lead levels, and in 1995, Canada's Federal-Provincial Committee on Environmental and Occupational Health showed that 5 to 10 percent of Canadian children living in urban areas also had elevated blood lead levels. A more recent study has shown that 50 percent of the children living near a lead and zinc smelter in Trail, British Columbia, have elevated blood lead levels.

As such data suggest, certain segments of the population are more likely to be exposed to lead than are others. Examples of occupations where exposure is likely to occur are lead mining and refining, plumbing and pipe fitting, auto repair (especially radiator repair), glass manufacturing, printing, battery manufacturing and recycling, construction work, firing-range instruction, plastic manufacturing, and working at a gas station. We also should be concerned about the lead content in paint, soil, or dust near roadways or lead-painted homes, plastic window blinds, garden hoses, plumbing leachate (from pipes or solder), ceramic ware, and lead-core candlewicks. Hobbies such as glazed pottery making, target shooting at firing ranges, lead soldering, preparing lead shot and fishing sinkers, stained glass making, painting, and car or boat repair also call for wariness, as do some kinds of folk remedies, children's toys, costume jewelry, and cosmetics (including lipsticks).

Health Problems Related to Lead

Lead is readily absorbed through the gastrointestinal and respiratory tracts. In adults, 20 to 70 percent of ingested lead and 100 percent of inhaled lead are absorbed by the body. Children between nine months to three years of age absorb lead five to ten times more effectively than adults, which makes them especially vulnerable. The major source of lead poisoning in children is contaminated dust and soil, which they ingest. Children living in older, deteriorated houses or houses undergoing renovations can be at risk as well.

Blood lead concentrations, even if they are below the current value considered acceptable (10ug/dl), have been linked to cognitive deficits in children, and these can persist into adulthood. There is strong evidence also linking low-level lead exposure early in life to later deficits in school performance, such as attention problems, aggressiveness, and antisocial or delinquent behavior. There is, therefore, persuasive evidence that low-level lead exposure causes persistent impairments of learning and other cognitive tasks.

The September 2006 issue of the journal *Circulation* contained a key research article on the impact of lead toxicity on the health of the general population. The researchers followed a group of 14,000 people over twelve years and studied the effect of lead on all causes of death. They found that even low blood lead levels (previously thought to be safe) were significantly associated with a higher incidence of heart attacks and strokes. They concluded that, "despite the marked decrease in blood lead levels over the past three decades, environmental lead exposures remain a significant determinant of cardiovascular mortality in the general population, constituting a major public health problem."[6]

If lead is not eliminated, it settles in the bones and is then released back into the body. In conditions where bones deteriorate, such as pregnancy[7] and osteoporosis from aging or prolonged immobilization, a greater release of lead occurs. It is now also recognized that when people are deficient in iron, they absorb more lead through their gastrointestinal tracts.

Lead is toxic to many tissues in our bodies, especially to the kidneys, which can be seriously damaged or fail altogether. Lead can also damage the nervous system, resulting in cognitive dysfunction, behavioral disturbances, depression, anxiety, and peripheral nerve damage. The cardiovascular system is also vulnerable to lead poisoning, which can result in an increased incidence of heart attacks and high blood pressure. Reproductive problems, a higher incidence of miscarriage, and low sperm counts can also be caused by exposure to lead, as can problems with the production of red blood cells, resulting in anemia. Common symptoms of lead toxicity include abdominal pain, joint pain, muscle pain, fatigue, irritability, difficulty in concentrating, and weakness of the limbs.

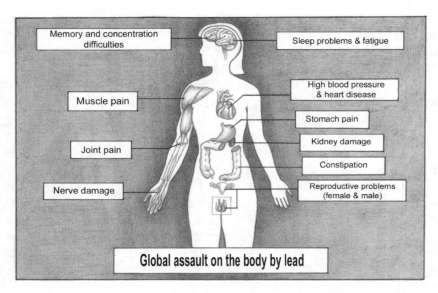

Figure 7.1 Global Assault on Body by Lead

Whole blood lead levels are the standard way to screen for lead toxicity, but if the exposure is not acute, blood lead levels can be low, even though the body's actual burden of lead is high. Two main methods are used to determine the results of low-level exposure. The first, which we use frequently in our clinic, measures urinary lead excretion after intravenous administration of the chelating agent EDTA (calcium ethlenediamine tetraacetic acid). The second is the use of Kappa x-ray fluorescence, which measures the lead deposited in bones.

The first thing to focus on in the treatment of lead toxicity is eliminating the source of exposure. Chelation therapy[8] can then be administered, using either intravenous EDTA, oral Penicillamine, or oral DMSA. Studies show that for people with high blood pressure or whose kidneys are not functioning well, the administration of intravenous EDTA chelation therapy is especially beneficial because it helps to improve kidney function.[9] I have also found that when people are given EDTA chelation therapy, their blood pressure often improves, a fact that may be related to the removal of lead. Another strategy, especially pertinent to the treatment of children, is to make sure that an iron deficiency is not present. If it is, the first step is to introduce iron-rich foods or to supplement with iron. If a child is low in iron, the body will tend to hold onto lead, making it more difficult to excrete.

Over the years we have treated thousands of people with elevated lead. Tom's case is a characteristic example.

Tom's Case

Tom, a sixty-year-old businessman, attended one of my community lectures and approached me afterwards to express concern about his health. At fifty-nine years of age, Tom had been diagnosed with Type II diabetes mellitus, which he was able to control with diet and exercise, so he had not developed any of the known complications. Since his teenage years he also had suffered from a chronic lack of energy that prevented him from performing vigorous exercise, although he was able to walk at a moderate pace for half an hour approximately five days per week. Because of his fatigue, his family doctor checked his testosterone level, which was low, but several injections of testosterone made no difference to his condition.

Tom also had problems with osteoarthritis of his knees. He had no problems with blood pressure, and he had given up smoking cigarettes when he was thirty-five years old. His cholesterol had never been elevated. When I asked about exposure to toxic substances, I learned that Tom had worked at a service station for two years, where he had significant exposure to leaded gasoline. Also, he had spent a lot of recreational time with motorboats, which would also have exposed him to leaded gasoline.

At fifty-six years old, Tom had most of his mercury amalgams removed. Because of his British heritage (see more about this in Chapter 9), together with his low testosterone level, diabetes, and arthritis, I advised him that he should be screened for iron overload. And because of his history of exposure to leaded gasoline, I recommended an EDTA challenge test.

My examination of Tom revealed many changes in his skin caused by sun exposure in the past. His blood pressure was excellent. There was no evidence of complications from diabetes mellitus. His right knee had changes compatible with chronic osteoarthritis. I ordered some tests, which showed that his fasting blood sugar was borderline elevated (5.9 mmol/L, with normal being 3.3-6.0). The test to look at blood sugar control over three months (Hb A1c) was good at 5.7 percent (with normal being less than 7 percent). He had no excessive protein in his urine, and his homocysteine, highly sensitive C-reactive protein, cholesterol indices, and chemistry reports were well within normal limits. However, the picture changed when we measured Tom's ferritin (the storage form of iron) and transferrin (the carrier protein for iron in the blood). His ferritin level was high (636 microgram/L, with normal being 30-300). His transferrin saturation was borderline elevated (55 percent, with normal being 20-55 percent). His serum iron was in the higher range of normal (28 micromol/L, with normal being 10-33). Genetic testing showed that he was homozygous for the C282Y genetic mutation for hemochromatosis, which means that he had a copy of this mutation from each of his parents. (See more about this in Chapter 9). Finally, an EDTA chelation challenge test showed a very elevated lead level (23 micrograms, with normal being less than 5). His mercury was mildly elevated (5.5, with normal being less than 3), and nickel also was elevated (20, with normal being less than 10). (see Figure 7.2)

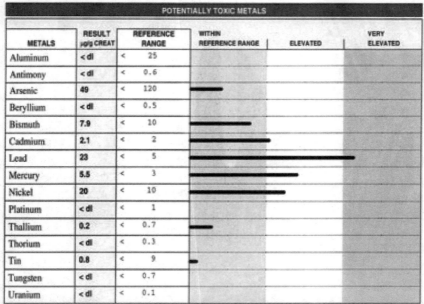

URINE TOXIC METALS

POTENTIALLY TOXIC METALS

METALS	RESULT µg/g CREAT	REFERENCE RANGE		WITHIN REFERENCE RANGE	ELEVATED	VERY ELEVATED
Aluminum	< dl	<	25			
Antimony	< dl	<	0.6			
Arsenic	49	<	120			
Beryllium	< dl	<	0.5			
Bismuth	7.9	<	10			
Cadmium	2.1	<	2			
Lead	23	<	5			
Mercury	5.5	<	3			
Nickel	20	<	10			
Platinum	< dl	<	1			
Thallium	0.2	<	0.7			
Thorium	< dl	<	0.3			
Tin	0.8	<	9			
Tungsten	< dl	<	0.7			
Uranium	< dl	<	0.1			

CREATININE

	RESULT mg/dL	REFERENCE RANGE	2SD LOW	1SD LOW	MEAN	1SD HIGH	2SD HIGH
Creatinine	19	45- 225					

SPECIMEN DATA

Comments:
Date Collected:	10/7/2004	Method: ICP-MS		Collection Period:	timed: 3 hours
Date Received:	10/8/2004	<dl: less than detection limit		Volume:	1700 ml
Date Completed:	10/11/2004	Provoking Agent: EDTA		Provocation:	POST PROVOCATIVE

Toxic metals are reported as µg/g creatinine to account for urine dilution variations. **Reference ranges are representative of a healthy population under non-challenge or non-provoked conditions.** No safe reference levels for toxic metals have been established.

V10.00

©DOCTOR'S DATA, INC. • ADDRESS: 3755 Illinois Avenue, St. Charles, IL 60174-2420 • CLIA ID NO: 14D0646470 • MEDICARE PROVIDER NO: 148463

Figure 7.2

URINE TOXIC METALS

POTENTIALLY TOXIC METALS

METALS	RESULT μg/g CREAT	REFERENCE RANGE	WITHIN REFERENCE RANGE	ELEVATED	VERY ELEVATED
Aluminum	< dl	< 25			
Antimony	< dl	< 0.6			
Arsenic	15	< 120	▬		
Beryllium	< dl	< 0.5			
Bismuth	< dl	< 10			
Cadmium	1.8	< 2	▬▬▬▬		
Lead	6.5	< 5	▬▬▬▬▬▬		
Mercury	0.5	< 3	▬		
Nickel	14	< 10	▬▬▬▬▬▬		
Platinum	< dl	< 1			
Thallium	0.2	< 0.7	▬▬		
Thorium	< dl	< 0.3			
Tin	0.7	< 9	▬		
Tungsten	0.06	< 0.7	▬		
Uranium	< dl	< 0.1			

CREATININE

	RESULT mg/dL	REFERENCE RANGE	2SD LOW	1SD LOW	MEAN	1SD HIGH	2SD HIGH
Creatinine	64	45- 225		▬▬▬▬▬▬			

SPECIMEN DATA

Comments:

Date Collected:	2/10/2005	Method: ICP-MS		Collection Period:	timed: 3 hours
Date Received:	2/14/2005	<dl: less than detection limit		Volume:	1100 ml
Date Completed:	2/15/2005	Provoking Agent: EDTA		Provocation:	POST PROVOCATIVE

Toxic metals are reported as μg/g creatinine to account for urine dilution variations. **Reference ranges are representative of a healthy population under non-challenge or non-provoked conditions.** No safe reference levels for toxic metals have been established.

V10.00

©DOCTOR'S DATA, INC. • ADDRESS: 3755 Illinois Avenue, St. Charles, IL 60174-2420 • CLIA ID NO: 14D0646470 • MEDICARE PROVIDER NO: 148453

Figure 7.3

Tom's treatment consisted of weekly phlebotomies to reduce his iron overload and EDTA chelation therapy to remove his toxic burden of lead and other metals. He was also instructed to decrease his intake of iron rich foods and limit his intake of vitamin C (vitamin C increases the absorption of iron). I also suggested that he contact the hemochromatosis society and advise his family members also to be tested for hemochromatosis. After nineteen phlebotomies, Tom's ferritin level had dropped from 636 to 28 mcg/L (the goal was to achieve a level of less than 50). After thirty treatments with EDTA chelation therapy, a challenge test showed a lead level of 6.5. His mercury level had also dropped to 0.5, and his nickel level had decreased to 14. (see Figure 7.3)

The main improvement Tom noticed as a result of these treatments was an increase in energy and well-being. His blood sugars continue to be well controlled, and he plans to continue with maintenance EDTA chelation therapy once a month. He will continue to have his ferritin level tested every three months, with phlebotomies performed as needed, so that his ferritin can be maintained at less than 50.

Case Discussion

Referring to the TILT Phenomenon, we can see that on the right side of the balance Tom was genetically predisposed to accumulating too much iron from his food, and by the time he reached sixty years of age, his iron storage was very high. Also, although his mercury amalgams were removed when he was fifty-six, he had been accumulating mercury for several decades. Furthermore, his long-term exposure to leaded gasoline reflected in a high level of lead in his first EDTA challenge test. These factors combined to tilt the balance towards the right, compromising Tom's health at the cellular level. With the removal of lead, iron, and other metals, the balance has now shifted towards the positive, and Tom has laid a good foundation for better health and quality of life during his retirement years.

As is frequently the case with patients at our clinic, Tom's illness had more than one cause, and we had to design his treatment accordingly. Both lead and iron were removed from his body, and he would not have regained good health had both tasks not been accomplished. I will have more to say about iron in Chapter 9; for now, Tom's case illustrates the harmful effects of lead toxicity and the effectiveness of chelation therapy in removing it.

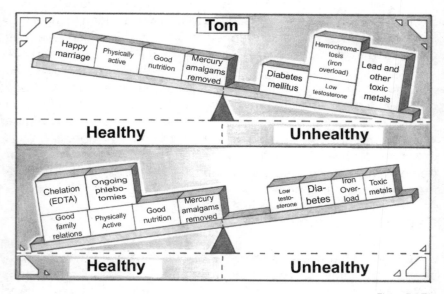

Figure 7.4 Tom

[1] Toxicological Profile For Lead, U.S. Department of Health and Human Services, Public Health Service, Agency for Toxic Substances and Disease Registry. 1999; 1-338. http://www.atsdr.cdc.gov.

[2] Priority List of Hazardous Substances, U.S. Department of Health and Human Services, www.atsdr.cdc.gov/cercla/05list.html

[3] Krantz A, Dorevitch S. Metal exposure and common chronic diseases: a guide for the clinician. Dis Mon. 2004 May; 50(5): 220-62.

[4] Sanborn MD, Abelsohn A, Campbell M, Weir E., Identifying and managing adverse environmental health effects: 3. Lead exposure. CMAJ. 2002 May 14; 166(10): 1287-92. Review.

[5] Lanphear BP, Hornung R, Ho M, Howard CR, Eberly S, Knauf K. Environmental lead exposure during early childhood. J Pediatr. 2002 Jan; 140(1): 40-7.

[6] Menke A, Muntner P, Batuman V, Silbergeld EK, Guallar E. Blood lead below 0.48 micromol/L (10 microg/dL) and mortality among U.S. adults. Circulation. 2006 Sep 26; 114(13):1388-94. Epub 2006 Sep 18.

[7] Whittaker S., Lead exposure in radiator repair workers: a survey of Washington State radiator repair shops and review of occupational lead exposure registry data. J Occup Environ Med. 2003 Jul; 45(7):724-33.

[8] Chelate is derived from the Greek word chele referring to the claw of a crab. The pincer-like binding action of certain chemical agents (natural or manmade), to metal ions is known as chelation. There are a variety of chelating agents available for therapeutic use.

[9] Lin JL, Lin-Tan DT, Li YJ, Chen KH, Huang YL. Low-level environmental exposure to lead and progressive chronic kidney diseases. Am J Med. 2006 Aug;119(8):707.e1-9.

Arsenic - Fit for Murder

Arsenic is a metal widely distributed in the earth's crust. In its natural form it is a steel-gray color, and it often binds with oxygen, chlorine, and sulfur to form inorganic arsenic compounds. By contrast, when it combines with carbon or hydrogen, organic arsenic is produced, which in general is less harmful than the inorganic kind.

Most arsenic compounds exist in the form of a white powder that, when dissolved, has no taste or odor; consequently, we cannot be directly aware of its presence in food, water, or air.[1] For this reason, arsenic was once the poison of choice for committing murder. Recently, I attended the theater production of *Arsenic and Old Lace,* a delightful comedy written in the 1940s about two elderly widows who run a boarding house. They systematically poison many of the men who come for overnight stays by offering them wine that has been laced with arsenic. The old ladies knew what they were doing; the men enjoyed the wine and did not taste the poison.

Today, forensic investigative abilities have made arsenic more difficult to use as a poison without being discovered. A recently published case involves a waitress who behaved much like the elderly widows in *Arsenic and Old Lace,* except that the waitress was quickly found out.[2] Her murderous activities were discovered when a forty-five-year-old traveling salesman was hospitalized with unexplained weakness and weight loss. He had also been hospitalized several times previously without a diagnosis being found. A pathologist then noticed multiple bands of transverse lines across the man's fingernails. When tests were conducted and arsenic was found, the physician recalled a similar recent case involving another traveling salesman who also showed signs of weakness and weight loss. Upon further investigation, the two men were discovered to have had similar sales territories. The second had died of unexplained causes, and his body was exhumed and tested. Arsenic again was found, and a subsequent criminal investigation discovered that both men ate regularly at the same department store lunch counter when they were in the same town, and both were served by the same waitress.

Because fingernails grow at a rate of approximately 0.1-0.15 mm per day, a rough estimate of when the first salesman visited the lunch counter was determined by measuring the distance between the telltale lines on his fingernails (technically known as "Mee's Lines"). The distance between the lines corresponded very well to his visits, and when the first salesman eventually died, the waitress was arrested and convicted of the double murder. As this disturbing story makes clear, arsenic is a deadly poison, and we can be adversely affected by it without our knowledge. This is no less the case if our exposure comes from natural sources rather than by the designs of a murderer.

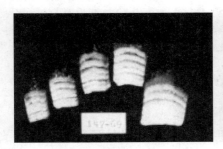 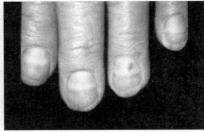

Mee's Lines

For instance, because arsenic is found throughout the earth's crust, it is a natural contaminant of groundwater. Consequently, arsenic can be present in our drinking water in varying degrees, depending on location.[3] Also, industrial processes such as mining, smelting, and coal-fired production of electric power can pump arsenic directly into rivers or into the air. In the air, it can travel great distances, coming down into waterways or onto the ground from where it is carried by rain into the groundwater. The seriousness of this issue was demonstrated in a recently published article in the *Canadian Medical Association Journal* entitled "Arsenic Threat Reaching Global Dimensions." Scientists have estimated that in recent decades approximately 140 million people worldwide have been exposed to excessive levels of arsenic in drinking water, and the situation is projected to become much worse.[4]

About 90 per cent of industrially produced arsenic is used to preserve wood from rot and decay. The preservative is CCA (chromated copper arsenate), and the treated wood is described as "pressure-treated." Arsenic has also been used as a pesticide, primarily on cotton fields and in orchards, although *inorganic* arsenic compounds are no longer permitted for use in agriculture. However, *organic* arsenicals, such as cacodylic acid, DSMA (disodium methylarsenate), and MSMA (monosodium methylarsenate) are still used as pesticides, principally on cotton. The residue from these applications is readily washed into rivers, lakes, and underground water supplies, and it should come as no surprise that arsenic is common in groundwater across the United States. Arsenic is also used in alloys and in the manufacture of lead-acid batteries for automobiles.

The main problem with the use of CCA for treating wood is that the arsenic gradually leaches out and accumulates in the soil.[5] A recent study[6] shows that soil samples taken from beneath CCA-treated wood decks are, on average, twenty times more contaminated with arsenic than soil samples taken from a farther distance. A serious problem arises when children play in the soil underneath pressure-treated wooden decks, or when they play on playground equipment built from pressure-treated wood. Although arsenic does not penetrate through the skin, it is rapidly absorbed if ingested from contaminated fingers.

A further problem arises if vegetables are grown in soil that is in close proximity to pressure-treated wood structures; arsenic from this soil is easily taken up by the vegetables and then consumed. Arsenic can also be found in the air in workplaces such as battery shops, mines, smelters, coal-burning electric power plants, or hazardous waste sites. It is also used in insecticides such as arsenate trioxide, which is found, for instance, in ant killers, and people have become severely ill from the accidental ingestion of these products.[7]

Arsenic is also found in commercially raised chickens. For many years, commercial chicken feed has contained arsenic in the form of roxarsone[8], which is supposed to promote growth, kill parasites that could cause diarrhea, and improve the pigmentation of the meat. It is true that roxarsone (a form of organic arsenic) is relatively benign, but when converted into an inorganic form, the arsenic in this product becomes highly toxic. Such a conversion from organic to inorganic occurs within the chicken itself, and subsequently, when chicken manure is spread on the land, it contaminates the soil and groundwater. Chicken manure is also made into fertilizer for use on commercial vegetable farms, home gardens, and lawns. It has been demonstrated that higher levels of arsenic are found in drinking water in areas where chicken manure is spread, as compared to drinking water in locations where no chicken manure is present.

If inorganic arsenic fumes are inhaled, a person can experience a sore throat or an irritation of the lungs.[9] Chronic low-level ingestion of inorganic arsenic can lead to nausea, vomiting, abnormal heart rhythms, high blood pressure, lowered production of red and white blood cells, damage to the lining of blood vessels, a sensation of "pins and needles" in the extremities, and reduced cognitive abilities (especially in children). Also, the skin can become a darker color, and there can be the appearance of what looks like corns or warts on the palms of the hands and soles of the feet. As we have seen, horizontal lines (Mee's Lines) can occur on the fingernails.

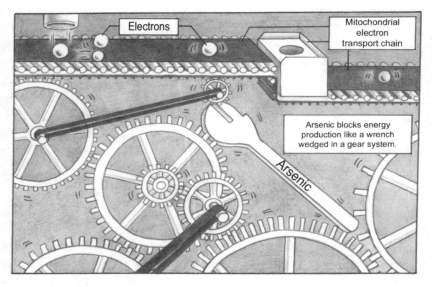

Figure 8.1 The Negative Impact of Arsenic on Celllular Energy Production

Numerous studies show that arsenic is a carcinogen, associated with cancers of the lung, skin, kidney, bladder, prostate, and liver. For instance, a recently published article in the *Journal of the National Cancer Institute*[10] shows that the degree of chromosomal damage in arsenic-associated bladder cancer is directly linked to the concentration of arsenic in the drinking water.

However, arsenic now can be detected easily by analysis of hair or nails, which can show the degree and extent of long-term exposure. Recent contamination can also be detected by analysis of the urine. Various chelating agents can be used to draw arsenic from the body, and it is then excreted through the urine.

John's Case

John was a fifty-eight-year-old retired heavy equipment operator who had a fifteen-year history of stiffness in his knee and ankle joints, a sensation of tightness of the skin in his lower limbs, as well as decreased sensation in both feet. He experienced cramps in his lower leg muscles approximately twice per week at night. The only medication he was taking was Lipitor® for high cholesterol. He also experienced occasional gout attacks in his feet if he consumed too much alcohol or protein. He noticed that during the last few years he had developed intolerance to cold, and he noticed that his balance was not as it should be. He did not have much exposure to mercury from amalgams because he had complete extraction of his teeth when he was eighteen years old, following an accident.

Several years before I met him, John had seen a naturopathic physician, who conducted a hair analysis that showed elevated levels of copper, selenium, mercury, and manganese. John had stopped smoking at forty-five years old, and he had one or two alcoholic drinks per day. He had a very bad family history for heart attacks: his father, all of his paternal uncles, and his paternal grandfather had died in their sixties from this cause. Consequently, John had recently undergone a treadmill test, which was normal. He told me that at work he had a lot of exposure to metals and chemicals. He also did all of his own mechanical work, which exposed him to various greases containing lead and arsenic. He was also exposed to leaded gasoline. He had spent a lot of time working with pressure-treated wood, and as a hobby, over several years he made his own lead bullets for black powder guns.

When I examined John, he appeared well, and his pulse and blood pressure were excellent. He had a few nonspecific changes in his fingernails, and he had vertical creases in his earlobes (which are often associated with coronary artery disease). He had a full set of dentures. His reflexes, however, were almost absent, and he had decreased sensation in his feet. He had difficulty walking heel-and-toe (as if walking on a tightrope), and when I asked him to stand with one foot directly in front of the other with his eyes closed, he fell over.

I performed a number of laboratory tests, including iron indices, homocysteine, highly sensitive C-reactive protein, thyroid indices, copper indices, kidney function tests, cholesterol indices, and the usual chemistry tests. These were all well within the normal ranges. I also suggested that we perform an EDTA chelation challenge test because of John's previous exposure to metals. He declined, but he wanted to proceed with a trial of EDTA chelation therapy. His cardiac treadmill test was negative, but because of his family history, I suggested that he consider getting an ultrafast CT scan of his coronary arteries (a reliable and noninvasive screening test for coronary artery disease).

Dietary instructions were reviewed, a nutritional supplement protocol was prescribed, and John began EDTA chelation treatments twice weekly. After fifteen treatments, both he and his wife noticed a remarkable improvement in his mood. His energy increased significantly, and his joints were more flexible, less swollen, and markedly less painful. The numb spots on his lower legs and feet disappeared, and for the first time in years he was able to feel the floor with the soles of his feet.

At this point, John agreed to have the EDTA chelation challenge test. The results showed an extremely high level of arsenic (500 mcg, with normal being less than 120). His cadmium level was also elevated (3.3, with normal being less than 2), as was his lead level (19, with normal being less than 5) and his nickel level (20, with normal being less than 10). John's arsenic level was one of the highest that I have observed, and when I questioned him further, I discovered that for many years he had consumed partially filtered well water. He also had a lot of exposure to pressure-treated wood.

John decided to get the ultrafast CT scan of his coronary arteries, but because there are no electron-beam computed tomography units in Canada, I referred him to a hospital in Seattle, Washington. His results were once again disturbing. The ultrafast CT scan calculates the amount of calcium in the lining of coronary arteries. This measurement is significant because the calcium level correlates 100 percent with the amount of plaque present.[11] People who have mild plaque in their arteries would have a calcium score of 100 or less. John's score was 3,910, discovered in twenty-two different sites.

Case Discussion

On reviewing his case according to the TILT Phenomenon model, we can see how John built up a burden of heavy metals over many years. He exhibited several symptoms and signs of heavy metal toxicity, but after fifteen treatments of EDTA chelation therapy he showed marked improvement in these symptoms and felt better than he had in a long time. John's very high levels of arsenic are especially notable, and it is a moot point whether or not arsenic contributed to his significant coronary artery disease. The plan is to continue with EDTA chelation therapy until the levels of toxic metals are down as far as we can get them. And so, John's story continues.

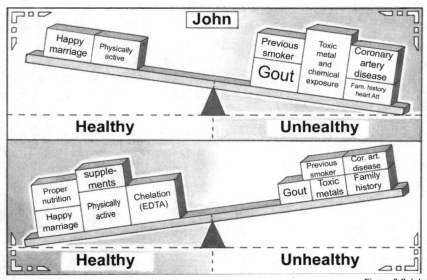

Figure 8.2 John

[1] Toxicological Profile for Arsenic, U.S. Department of Health and Human Services, Public Health Service, Agency for Toxic Substances and Disease Registry. 2000; 1-468. http://www. atsdr.cdc.gov.

[2] Daniel CR 3rd, Piraccini BM, Tosti A. The nail and hair in forensic science. J Am Acad Dermatol. 2004 Feb; 50(2): 258-61.

[3] Weir E., Arsenic and drinking water. CMAJ. 2002 Jan 8; 166(1): 69.

[4] Bagchi S. Arsenic threat reaching global dimensions. CMAJ. 2007 Nov 20; 177(11): 1344-1345.

[5] Sibbald B. Arsenic and pressure-treated wood: the argument moves to the playground. CMAJ. 2002 Jan 8; 166(1): 79.

[6] Stilwell DE, Gorny KD. Contamination of soil with copper, chromium, and arsenic under decks built from pressure treated wood. Bull Environ Contam Toxicol. 1997 Jan; 58(1): 22-9.

[7] Stephanopoulus DE, et al. Treatment and toxicokinetics of acute pediatric arsenic ingestion: danger of arsenic insecticides in children. Pediatr Crit Care Med. 2002 Jan; 3(1): 74-80.

[8] Hileman B. Arsenic in chicken production. A common feed additive adds arsenic to human food and endangers water supplies. Chemical and Engineering News. 2007 Apr 9; 85(15):34-35.

[9] Ibrahim D, et al. Heavy Metal Poisoning: Clinical Presentations and Pathophysiology. Clin Lab Med. 2006 Feb; 26: 67-97.

[10] Moore LE, Smith AH, Eng C, Kalman D, DeVries S, Bhargava V, Chew K, Moore D 2nd, Ferreccio C, Rey OA, Waldman FM. Arsenic-related chromosomal alterations in bladder cancer. J Natl Cancer Inst. 2002 Nov 20; 94(22): 1688-96.

[11] Forster BB, Isserow S. Coronary artery calcification and subclinical atherosclerosis: what's the score? BC Med J. 2005 May; 47(4): 181-187.

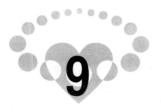

The Ironman

Yes, the Ironman® is an elite triathlon held in Kona, Hawaii, each year, and, no, this chapter is not about that triathlon. Instead, my topic in the following pages is iron overload, which can cause serious and even fatal health disorders. Yet, unlike mercury, lead, and arsenic, iron in itself is not necessarily harmful and, indeed, is required for healthy cellular function. The problem is that too little iron leads to a whole range of health problems, and too much iron leads to acceleration of the aging and degenerative processes. In my medical practice, I meet iron-men and iron-women all the time, partly because I screen almost everyone who comes through the door for hemochromatosis, which is a major cause of iron overload and also the most common inherited disorder in the Western world.[1]

Iron Metabolism and Hemochromatosis

Iron has a unique ability to accept and donate electrons, the energy currency on which our bodies work. Iron also is required in cells that bind oxygen, such as hemoglobin in red blood cells and myoglobinin in muscle cells. Without iron, oxygen cannot be delivered to the trillions of cells in our bodies; consequently, if iron levels are low, energy production will drop. Anyone who has suffered from iron deficiency anemia will recognize the many symptoms that accompany this condition: fatigue, cold intolerance, cognitive sluggishness, palpitations, a racing heart after slight exertion, and muscle weakness.

Healthy adult males have 3 to 4 grams of iron in their bodies, and women have slightly less. An average male adult absorbs and loses approximately 1 mg of iron per day, and a premenopausal woman loses approximately 2 mg per day. There is no effective means (other than menstruation) of excreting excess iron, and the balance is entirely dependent on the rate of absorption of iron across the intestinal wall. When we are healthy and our bodies are well adjusted, the cells lining our gastrointestinal tract simply stop absorbing excess iron from the food we eat. Conversely, when our bodies lack iron, more is absorbed. The HFE gene regulates this absorption, but if a mutation of this gene is inherited from each parent, then hemochromatosis will likely develop. This is a disorder in which control over the absorption of iron is lost so that most, if not all, ingested iron crosses into the body. One consequence is that the rate of oxidation (aging) speeds up dramatically. People of northwestern European descent stand a 1 in 6 chance of inheriting only one gene with the mutation and a 1 in 200 chance of inheriting two genes with the mutation. People of Irish descent stand a 1 in 4 chance of inheriting one gene with the mutation.

So far, two genetic mutations with a direct bearing on hemochromatois have been characterized: C282Y and H63D. Approximately 95 percent of those diagnosed with hemochromatosis have the C282Y mutation present, but only a small fraction of those who have the H63D mutation actually develop the disorder. Interestingly, not everybody who has the genetic mutations goes on to develop the syndrome, and researchers are looking into the possible significance of other genetic mutations which may also be associated with this disorder.

The main issue with hemochromatosis is that an excessive amount of free, or unbound iron in our tissues drives up the production of free radicals. You may remember from Chapter 3 that free radicals are highly reactive molecules that strip the electrons from molecules in close proximity. People with hereditary hemochromatosis gradually develop large deposits of iron in every major organ of the body (especially the liver, pancreas, and heart), and the resultant accelerated production of free radicals can cause widespread organ failure.

Clinical Manifestations

Most people with hemochromatosis have numerous symptoms. Just as mercury has been called "the great masquerader," so also excessive levels of iron can masquerade as other disorders, and the diagnosis is often missed. The classic presentation includes a bronze or gray skin pigmentation, liver disease, diabetes mellitus, and gonadal failure. Liver disease can include a wide range of problems including fibrosis, cirrhosis, and even cancer. Heart abnormalities such as dysrhythmias and enlargement of the heart muscle can occur. Painful swelling of the joints is also common and can easily be misdiagnosed as rheumatoid-like arthritis. Fatigue is also common, and early dementia can occur. Even more seriously, people afflicted with iron overload often have heart attacks beginning in their forties or fifties.

If hemochromatosis is suspected, the most reliable screening blood test is transferrin saturation. Any physician can order this test, and, if it is positive, other iron indices such as ferritin can be ordered, as well as genetic testing, which also is readily available. Liver biopsy was once the gold standard for this diagnosis, but has been largely superseded by genetic testing.

Once the diagnosis is made, treatment is relatively simple. Basically, excess iron is taken out, and too much iron is prevented from coming in. It is important to avoid consuming foods that are rich in iron, such as spinach and organ meats. It is also advisable to cut down on the excessive consumption of red meat, and large quantities of vitamin C should be avoided (especially when taken with food), because vitamin C increases the absorption of iron.

Excess iron can be removed by taking blood (phlebotomy) one pint at a time at weekly intervals until the ferritin levels have dropped to less than 50. This procedure can be repeated as frequently as is required. Also, an extract from rice bran, called phytic acid, can be taken orally. This product, IP6, is readily available in health food stores. Recently, an oral pharmaceutical iron-chelating product called Deferasirox came on the market. After approximately one year, it was taken off the market because too many people were dying of liver failure after taking it.

In our clinic, we often combine EDTA chelation therapy with the use of phlebotomies and dietary changes. We have observed that people often do much better when a chelating agent such as EDTA is used, because iron is probably not the only harmful metal present, and the removal of several metals at once has a greater positive impact at the cellular level.

Kevin's Case

Kevin was a fifty-eight-year-old disabled logger with several health problems including stable angina, diabetes mellitus, rheumatoid-like arthritis, and a generalized fatigue that was not relieved with rest.

Kevin's problems began when he underwent carpal tunnel syndrome repair at age fifty-three. During the procedure, he had a minor heart attack that resulted in extended hospitalization. During this time, tests revealed that Kevin's blood sugars were elevated. He was placed on oral medication for diabetes mellitus, as well as on nitroglycerin and a beta-blocker medication for his heart.

Over the next few years, Kevin noticed progressive pain, stiffness, and swelling in his knuckles, shoulders, knees, and ankles. He was referred to a rheumatologist who diagnosed a rheumatoid-like arthritis (previous blood tests were negative for actual rheumatoid arthritis). Kevin then was placed on a powerful drug to stop the inflammation in his joints; nevertheless, he was still unable to carry a bag of groceries because of the pain in his hands. Unfortunately, during the five years before I met Kevin, he developed angina (pain in his chest on exertion, relieved by rest or a nitroglycerin spray). He now was able to walk only half a block before the onset of symptoms.

In the past, Kevin had been generally healthy and very active, and he had enjoyed working as a logger. He was a nonsmoker, and his blood pressure had never been elevated. His cholesterol had always been in the normal range, though several relatives on his father's side had experienced heart attacks in their fifties and sixties. Mercury didn't seem to be an issue (partly because Kevin had all his teeth extracted several decades previously).

When I examined him, Kevin appeared tired and seemed older than his fifty-eight years. His skin was a pale gray color, he had mild chronic swelling of his knuckle joints, and he found it hard to elevate his arms above his shoulders. His knees also appeared chronically swollen. Otherwise, his examination was unremarkable.

I ordered iron indices and was somewhat taken aback at how high the levels were. Transferrin saturation was 65 percent, with normal being 20-55 percent. Ferritin (the storage form of iron) was 2600 ug/L, with normal being 30-300. Interestingly, Kevin's serum iron level was 20 umol/L, with normal being 10-33, so if I had ordered only his serum iron level, I would have missed the diagnosis.

Genetic studies were then ordered, and they revealed that Kevin was homozygous for the C282Y genetic mutation for hemochromatosis. This means that he inherited one mutation from each parent, so a diagnosis of hereditary hemochromatosis was made.

Kevin began weekly phlebotomy treatments, which removed 1 pint of blood each time. He tolerated this very well, and he then started on a weekly course of EDTA chelation therapy. After two months, he noticed that his energy had improved, and, more importantly, his angina symptoms were less frequent. He was now able to walk much farther before developing chest pain, and he used his sublingual nitroglycerin less often. As his treatments progressed, his blood sugars began to drop, and when his blood sugars stabilized within the normal range, he was able to discontinue his oral medication. Gradually, his joint symptoms began to lessen, and he was able to do various jobs around his property without suffering from joint inflammation. After about eight months of treatments, Kevin's ferritin level dropped to 70 ug/L, he was off all medication, and he was able to resume his active lifestyle. He even felt so well that he purchased a gas station and went into business. Kevin has continued with maintenance phlebotomies, and he has been enjoying his renewed health.

Case Discussion

In light of the TILT Phenomenon, it is clear that the toxic buildup of excessive iron in Kevin's body caused a tilt to the right, and Kevin went on a downward plunge, culminating in his heart attack during a surgical procedure. Despite trying to remain active, watching his diet, and taking numerous prescribed medications, he was unable to tilt his system back into balance. The intervention that saved his life was the diagnosis of hemochromatosis, followed by appropriate treatment. I should mention that his brother and sister were also tested, and both were found to be homozygous for the same mutation.

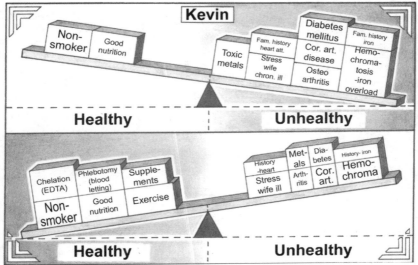

Figure 9.1 Kevin

If you are a person of northwestern European descent (especially if you are suffering from any of the above listed disorders such as heart disease, diabetes mellitus, arthritis, or severe fatigue), you should have your physician test you for transferrin saturation and also conduct other standard tests for iron. If these are positive, you should insist on genetic testing so that a diagnosis of hemochromatosis is not missed in your case. If you do happen to test positive, then your children and siblings should also be tested, because early treatment can prevent serious consequences.[2]

---

[1] Heeney M, Andrews N. Iron homeostasis and inherited iron overload disorders: an overview. Hematol Oncol Clin North Am. 2004 Dec; 18(6): 1379

[2] Very good and easy-to-read information can be found at www.ironichealth.com.

10

POP Culture

POPs: What Are They?

The pop culture that I will be discussing in this chapter has nothing to do with teenage trends in music, but rather with Persistent Organic Pollutants, or POPs. These are chemicals containing carbon (hence organic), and they accumulate in the fat of living organisms. They increase in quantity as they go up the food chain, and they also persist in the environment that they pollute. Most POPs are volatile, which means they can travel in the air, even thousands of miles, before they settle. For instance, the Inuit of Nunavik in northern Canada consume the fat of seals, beluga, and narwhal whales. These people have high body burdens of POPs,[1] which shows how POPs can affect people living far away from the source of the chemicals. POPs resist degradation (breaking down) and can take as long as a hundred years to dissipate.

Few environmental issues have aroused more public concern than the effects of POPs on the general population, and especially on the health and welfare of children. Despite the volume of scientific literature published, this topic remains highly controversial because enormous amounts of money are at stake. Approximately 100,000 manmade chemicals have been invented since World War II, and the costs of producing and marketing these chemicals are immense.[2]

Before World War II, pesticides did not exist. They were developed for use in combat as defoliants and nerve gases. Phenoxyherbicides such as 2,4-D were designed to destroy Japanese rice crops and were later used in Agent Orange, which was deployed in Vietnam to defoliate large areas of jungle. Following World War II, these chemicals were used in agricultural production and to spray entire neighborhoods to eradicate mosquitoes.

Since the 1950s, epidemiologists have become increasingly concerned about the health effects of exposure to POPs. Studies of wildlife communities demonstrate reproductive, developmental, endocrine, immunologic, and carcinogenic effects, with high rates of malformed genitalia, aberrant mating behavior, sterility, and cancer, as well as immune system and thyroid dysfunction.[3] Epidemiologists in the United States have noticed a rise in the incidence of NHL (Non-Hodgkin's Lymphoma), especially in agricultural areas. This high incidence correlates well with pesticide use and has caused some researchers to see a link between POPs and the disease. In 1962, Rachel Carson's book, *Silent Spring,* brought this important issue into public awareness,[4] and in 1996, T. Colborn's *Our Stolen Future*[5] effectively delivered an urgent message of a similar kind.

In 1996, a number of governments participated in the Intergovernmental Forum on Chemical Safety, where they agreed upon a list of twelve POPs to be eliminated from the environment. These twelve have been dubbed "The Dirty Dozen." In 2001, the United Nations Environment Program sponsored the Binding Convention on Persistent Organic Pollutants and called for an immediate ban on eleven of these twelve worst culprits. The entire Dirty Dozen are listed below in Table 1, together with their most common sources.[6] It should be noted that DDT is still being used in developing countries to control mosquitoes, with a view to preventing malaria.

TABLE 1 – Environmental and Dietary Sources of Persistent Organic Pollutants (The "Dirty Dozen")

Type	Environmental sources	Examples of dietary sources
Dioxins, furans	By-products of petrochemical industry and chlorine bleaching in pulp and paper mills; hospital and municipal incinerators	Meat, poultry, and dairy products; sport fish (e.g., lake trout, salmon, walleye); wildlife (e.g., waterfowl and waterfowl eggs, muskrat, otter, moose, deer)
PCBs	"Fire resistant" synthetic products made before 1977; old electrical equipment; leaky containers in PCB disposal sites	Great Lakes fish (e.g., lake trout, salmon); arctic marine mammals, breast milk
Aldrin	Pesticide used against insects in the soil and to protect crops, such as corn and potatoes	Dairy products; meat; fish; oils and fats; potatoes and root vegetables
Chlordane	Broad-spectrum contact insecticide used on vegetables, grains, maize, oilseed, potatoes, sugar cane, beets, fruits, nuts, cotton, and jute	Use has been severely restricted, so food does not appear to be a major pathway of exposure; air may be a pathway because of continued use in termite control (in the United States)
DDT	Pesticide widely used during World War II to protect soldiers and civilians against diseases spread by insects	Fish; dairy products; fat of cattle, hogs, poultry and sheep; eggs; vegetables

Type	Environmental sources	Examples of dietary sources
Dieldrin	Insecticide used to control insects in soil	Same as for aldrin
Endrin	Foliar (leaf) insecticide used on field crops, such as cotton	Current dietary exposure thought to be minimal because of restricted use
Heptachlor	Nonsystemic stomach and contact insecticide used to control insects in soil	Detected in the blood of U.S. and Australian cattle in 1990; current dietary exposure thought to be minimal because of restricted use
HCB	Fungicide used for seed treatment	HCB-treated grain; current dietary exposure thought to be very low because of severely restricted use
Mirex	Stomach insecticide used to control ants, termites, and mealy bugs	Meat, fish, wild game; marine bird eggs; sea mammals
Toxaphene	Contact insecticide used primarily on cotton, cereal, grains, fruits, nuts, and vegetables; used to control tick and mites in livestock	Dietary exposure thought to be very low because of restricted use; however, there is a local problem with some fish in Lake Superior

Note: PCBs = polychlorinated biphenyls, DDT = dichlorodiphenyltrichloroethane, HCB = hexachlorobenzene

How POPs Affect You

Epidemiological evidence suggests that the health effects of POPs in humans are similar to those in animals in the same range of exposures. Specifically, studies demonstrate that POPs have negative effects on neurodevelopmental, thyroid, estrogen, and immune function.[1] Exposure to commonly used pesticides such as pheonxyherbicides, organophosphates, carbamates, and pyrethrins is also shown to be associated with adverse health effects. For example, studies show that mothers who ate large amounts of fish caught in Lake Michigan, which had been contaminated with PCBs (polychlorinated biphenyls), had lower birth rates. Also, their babies had smaller head circumferences and shorter attention spans than babies whose mothers did not eat fish from that source. The affected children were monitored over a period of eleven years; they continued to do poorly in a range of skills and developmental tests, which indicated deficits in general intellectual functioning, short and long-term memory, and attention span.[2]

Other studies demonstrate that higher levels of PCBs adversely affect the brain development of unborn children. For instance, there is evidence of altered gender-typical play behavior in boys and girls, as well as poor impulse control of the kind frequently found in children with attention deficit hyperactivity disorder (ADHD).[3] Furthermore, the carcinogenic effects of certain POPs are also well demonstrated. We now know that Triazine herbicides increase breast cancer risk; carbamate and phenoxyherbicides increase lung cancer risk; the use of indoor insecticides increases the risk for brain cancer as well as lymphocytic leukemia in children.

Flame-retardants should also be mentioned in this context. Although there are 175 listed types of flame-retardants, the brominated ones (BFRs) make up the majority. Tetrabromobisphenol A is the most widely used, and studies demonstrate that it is toxic to the liver, the immune system, and the nervous system. It also disrupts hormones and has estrogen-like properties, as well as a toxic effect on thyroid function.[4] There is speculation that earlier puberty in women and the feminization of men are a result of these types of POPs in the environment. A study of people living in the remote Faroe Islands shows that the level of PBDEs (polybrominated diphenyl ethers) is rising, and, alarmingly, the concentration of PBDEs in the breast milk of Faroe Island mothers tripled between 1987 and 1999.[5]

One of the most comprehensive assessments of the effects of POPs is the *Systematic Review of Pesticide Human Health Effects* [6]. The authors conclude that exposure to all the commonly used pesticides – such as phenoxyherbicides, organophosphates, carbamates, and pyrethrins – causes adverse health effects. Thus, triazine herbicides increase breast cancer risk; carbamate and phenoxyherbicide increase lung cancer risk; organophosphates sprayed during pregnancy result in deterioration of the placenta; indoor use of insecticides is associated with brain cancer and acute lymphocytic leukemia in children; six pesticides (including 2,4-D and dicamba) are associated with infertility; fungicide exposure has positive associations with dermatitis; pyrethrins are associated with chronic psychiatric effects, chromosomal defects, intrauterine growth retardation, and rashes in licensed pet groomers; glyphosate and glufosinate have been associated with congenital malformations; and glyphosate is associated with late abortion if exposure occurs before conception.

Because of the wide range of commonly used home and garden products associated with adverse health effects, exposure to all pesticides should be avoided. Research shows that there is an increased risk of childhood acute lymphocytic leukemia when women use pesticides in the home and garden during pregnancy. Other adverse effects include an increased incidence of miscarriage, fetal death, infertility, and birth defects. Women who are contemplating pregnancy should therefore avoid using pesticides in their homes, gardens, and workplaces.

Children are highly vulnerable to pesticides, and many studies show an elevated cancer risk in children who have been exposed, either directly or indirectly. Children may be exposed directly through the use of pesticides on lawns, gardens, school playgrounds, and parks, or in the treatment of pets. But there is also an increased risk of brain cancer and kidney cancer in the offspring of occupationally exposed men, which suggests that indirect exposure can also be harmful. The elderly likewise can develop chronic neurological diseases such as Parkinson's disease, Amyotrophic Lateral Sclerosis (ALS), and Alzheimer's disease as a consequence of long-term pesticide exposure.[7]

We are currently able to characterize the risks for only a small number of the 100,000-plus POPs that have been released into our environment. Even if we were to limit our scrutiny to the 5,000 most prevalent (those produced in amounts greater than one million metric tons per year), it would be impossible to predict the effect on humans. There are incalculable combinations of chemicals, environmental breakdown molecules, and metabolites to be evaluated for safety, and we simply do not have enough information. Consequently, the phrase "no evidence of harmful effects" leaves the question open; in fact, there might well be very harmful effects, which we have not yet had sufficient time or opportunity to notice.[8]

I do not have any cases to discuss in this section, because virtually everyone who comes into my clinic has POPs present to some extent. Some, no doubt, have more in their systems than others, depending on their history of exposure and their ability to detoxify. The important route of excretion of these chemicals is through the liver detoxification pathways discussed in Chapter 5. Another important way to mobilize and excrete POPs is by regular use of a far infrared sauna, which is a gentle and safe tool to assist the detoxification process. However, as I have already suggested, the most important way to reduce contamination from POPs is to avoid being exposed to them.

[1] Ribas-Fito N et.al. Polychlorinated biphenyls (PCBs) and neurological development in children: a systematic review. J Epidemiol Community Health 2001; 55:537-46.

Brouwer A et.al. Interactions of persistent environmental organohalogens with the thyroid hormone system: mechanisms and possible consequences for animal and human health. Toxicol Ind Health 1998; 14:59-84.

Wade M. Human health and exposure to chemicals which disrupt estrogen, androgen and thyroid hormone physiology. Ottawa: Environmental and Occupational Toxicology Division, Environmental Health Directorate, Health Protection Branch, Health Canada. Available: www.hc-sc.gc.ca/ehp/ehd/bch/env_contaminants/endocrine.pdf (accessed 2002 May 13).

[2] Jacobson J, Jacobson S, Humphrey H. Effects of in utero exposure to polychlorinated biphenyls and related contaminants on cognitive function in young children. J Pediatr 1990; 116:38-45.

Jacobson J, Jacobson S, Humphrey H. Effects of exposure to PCBs and related compounds on growth and activity in children. Neurotoxicol Teratol 1990; 12:319-26.

Jacobson J, Jacobson S. Intellectual impairment in children exposed to polychlorinated biphenyls in utero. N Engl J Med 1996; 335:783-9.

[3] Vreugdenhil HJ, Slijper FM, Mulder PG, Weisglas-Kuperus N. Effects of perinatal exposure to PCBs and dioxins on play behavior in Dutch children at school age. Environ Health Perspect. 2002 Oct; 110(10):A593-8.

Stewart P, Fitzgerald S, Reihman J, Gump B, Lonky E, Darvill T, Pagano J, Hauser P. Prenatal PCB exposure, the corpus callosum, and response inhibition. Environ Health Perspect.2003 Oct; 111(13):1670-7.

[4] Birnbaum L S et.al. Brominated flame retardants: cause for concern? Environ Health Perspect 2004; 112:9-17.

[5] Fangstrom B, Strid A, Grandjean P, Weihe P, Bergman A. A retrospective study of PBDEs and PCBs in human milk from the Faroe Islands. Environ Health. 2005 Jul 14; 4(1):12

[6] Sandborn M et.al. Systematic review of pesticide human health effects. Ontario College of Family Physicians 2004:1-186. www.ocfp.on.ca

[7] Caban-Holt A, Mattingly M, Cooper G, Schmitt FA. Neurodegenerative memory disorders: a potential role of environmental toxins. Neurol Clin. 2005 May;23(2):485-521. Review.

[8] Shea KM. Protecting our children from environmental hazards in the face of limited data-a precautionary approach is needed. J Pediatr. 2004 Aug; 145(2):145-7.

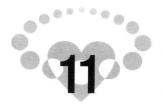

Electromagnetic Fields - Don't Be Overcharged

Most of us are exposed to the abnormal electromagnetic fields which have increased markedly in our environment as technology has progressed. As I pointed out in Chapter 2, each cell in our body is like an organism that needs to eat, drink, breathe, and detoxify itself by taking in nutrients and eliminating waste products across the cell membrane. The rate at which substances are exchanged across the cell membrane determines how efficiently the cell is working. In turn, the rate of exchange is dependent on the status of the membrane potential, which is the difference in the electrical charge on either side of the membrane.

Cell membrane potential is usually around 80 millivolts (mV), but when the cell's normal electrical function is impaired, the ion pumps and ionic channels in the membrane stop working. The cell then becomes electrically paralyzed and cannot eliminate its waste products. As a result, abnormal minerals and toxic substances accumulate and interfere with the cell's ability to heal itself and maintain normal function. Exposure to abnormal electromagnetic fields can cause this kind of disruption in the membrane potential, but the cell is able to detoxify once it is out of the range of the damaging electrical field.

In 2002, Dr. De-Kun Li, a reproductive epidemiologist, published a study of the effects of electromagnetic fields on pregnant women.[1] A total of 969 pregnant women were interviewed about known risk factors for miscarriage. They were then asked to wear a gauss meter for twenty-four hours. The magnetic field exposure was recorded every ten seconds, and a diary of the women's activities was kept. The overall rate of miscarriage in the group was 16 percent. Among women who were exposed to a peak magnetic field measuring less than 16 milligauss (mG), the miscarriage rate was 10.7 percent. The rate rose to 18.4 percent among women exposed to a peak magnetic field of 16 mG or greater. The association remained statistically significant after adjusting for thirty known risk factors for miscarriage and other potential confounders. The association was even stronger for miscarriages occurring at less than ten weeks' gestation.

Dr. Li speculates that external magnetic fields may increase the risk of miscarriage by interfering with internally generated fields inside fetal cells. These internal fields may play a role in cellular communication critical for fetal development, and they are affected by the external fields generated by such things as shavers, vacuum cleaners, electric vehicles (trams, trains and the like). Dr. Li especially recommends that in order to reduce magnetic field exposure to the fetus, pregnant women should not use hair dryers, and if they do, they should hold the dryer as far away from the abdomen as possible. Also, they should not stand next to a microwave oven when it is in operation.

Power companies usually have a service whereby customers can borrow or rent a gauss meter, which can be used to confirm whether or not a person is being exposed to abnormal electromagnetic fields.

Jane's Case

Jane was a 45-year-old married woman and mother of two adult sons. Other than chronic, intermittent inflammation of the eyes, she had been generally healthy and active until she and her husband moved into a brand new home, approximately two years before she first visited our clinic. Jane noticed that despite frequent cleaning she could not get rid of a fine layer of white dust that settled everywhere throughout her new house. She also noticed that her energy was gradually decreasing and her muscles and joints had become painful. Exposure to a variety of fumes, especially fresh newsprint, caused her to lose her voice, and she developed headaches, severe fatigue, and sudden impairments in the functioning of her mind. When she was out of her home, she began to feel slightly better. The family dog also became sick and vomited frequently, and after one year of living in the new home, the dog died. A careful inspection then revealed that the sealant coat on the cement floor in the basement of the house had been improperly applied and a constant off-gassing of material from the floor was picked up by the air intake of the heating system. This was corrected and the problem was supposedly fixed but Jane did not recover her health, and when she first visited our clinic she was living in a hotel room.

After talking to Jane for a brief time, I realized that the TILT Phenomenon was probably applicable in her case, and so I had her recount her medical history from childhood to the present. As a young child she had the usual mercury-preserved vaccinations, and her tonsils were removed. Later, she had a large number of mercury fillings placed in her teeth. However, her teeth were very brittle, and in her twenties she had most of them extracted; consequently, she now wore upper and lower dentures. As a young woman Jane began smoking several cigarettes per day. For many years she used chemical fertilizers on her lawns and plants. Due to very heavy menstrual periods, at twenty-six-years old she had a hysterectomy, with one ovary preserved. At thirty-years-old she developed uveitis, an inflammatory condition in her eyes. This was treated with oral prednisone (a powerful steroid drug) approximately four times a year, and she used steroid and anti-inflammatory eye drops daily. When she was thirty-six-years old, her gallbladder was removed through a laparoscope, and at thirty-nine she had saline breast implants placed. Two years later she had a disc removed in her lumbar spine, and subsequently she experienced chronic constipation, as well as bloating and gas after eating. At forty years of age, she took up a hobby making stained glass windows, thereby exposing herself to lead. Finally, when she moved into her new, toxic house, a tipping point was reached, after which her health declined rapidly.

On examining Jane, I noticed that she appeared tired, her skin was dry, and her voice would cut out at times. She explained to me that she was having a bad reaction to the paper on the examining table. She also had signs on her skin that her liver was stressed and not functioning as it should. She had the expected scars on her skin from the previously mentioned surgical procedures. Her balance was not as good as it should have been, but her laboratory tests were surprisingly normal, showing only a slight reaction of her immune system to her muscle cells.

I told Jane that she needed to quit smoking, and I described some ways in which she might go about doing this. I then prescribed an elimination diet (see Appendix B) and a medical food product called Ultra Clear Plus pH ®, which is designed to heal the lining of the gastrointestinal tract. This product also helps the liver to work efficiently as a detoxification organ balancing the phase 1 and phase 2 pathways (see Chapter 5) and excreting toxic elements through the bile into the bowel, and through the kidneys into the urine. Jane also began taking a high dose of probiotics (the friendly bacteria) and she used digestive enzymes with each meal. I recommended that she take magnesium glycinate, as well as a good dose of fish oil.

Within two weeks Jane was feeling much better, but, unfortunately, whenever she went back into her home she began to feel ill again. At this point I suspected there might be a problem with the electrical system in the new house. At our clinic we have a Graham-Stetzer meter so that patients can evaluate their homes and workplaces for dirty electrical fields. After evaluating their home, Jane's husband reported that most of the electrical outlets in the house were showing readings of 1300, with the average reading equal to 600 (normal should be less than 25). Jane and her husband placed approximately twenty Graham-Stetzer filters in the electrical outlets and, for the first time, Jane could enter her home without an adverse reaction. This was a great breakthrough in her case.

Recently, Jane reported to me that her denturist had given her a new partial plate for her lower jaw. She discovered that when she had the plate in her mouth she would react to wireless radio waves, but when she removed the plate she had no such reaction. Her denturist evaluated the partial plate and found a metal strip that was magnetically active. He revised the plate and she no longer reacts to wireless radio waves. I will continue to treat Jane with Neural Therapy for her scars (as discussed later in this chapter), testing for heavy metals and recommendations for diet and nutrition, until she has made a full recovery. I should mention that some of my patients get their breast implants carefully removed as they are potentially hazardous due to the release of silicone as well as chemicals from the plastics.

Case Discussion

Jane's exposure to toxic elements began as an infant with a series of mercury-preserved vaccines. She then had a large number of mercury amalgams placed in her teeth and also had her tonsils removed. She was a smoker and used chemical herbicides and fertilizers for many years. Many surgical procedures left her with scars that had the potential to be electrically active. Breast implants were a source of ongoing exposure to chemicals released from the plastic. She also had exposure to lead from working with stained glass windows. The final tipping point for Jane was the exposure to chemicals off-gassing from the improperly finished basement floor as well as the dirty electrical fields throughout her new home. The health restoration process started when she removed herself from the toxic house. Placing her on the elimination diet, adding the medical food product Ultra Clear Plus pH ®, probiotics, fish oil, and magnesium resulted in a marked improvement in the function of her own detoxification mechanisms. A major improvement occurred when the dirty electrical fields in her new home were neutralized with the Graham-Stetzer filters. There is still a lot of work left to do in her case. Nonetheless, Jane's story to date shows how rapidly an improvement in health can be achieved by simple detoxification methods.

Dirty Electricity

Most people do not realize that the electrical wiring in their homes or workplaces can be a source of harmful electromagnetic fields. Energy travels through space in the form of waves; we commonly refer to radio waves, microwaves, and sound waves. The characteristics of such waves can be measured accurately by using various pieces of equipment, and the typical shape of a wave of energy is seen in the figure below.

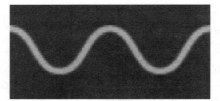

Figure 11.1

In this figure, we see a form that is clean and without distortion. Clean electricity produces a wave like this, but "dirty electricity" produces a distorted pattern, as in the figure below.

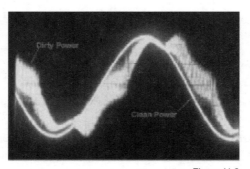

Figure 11.2

At least three sources of energy can distort normal wave forms and cause electrical waves to become "dirty." First, electrical appliances and gadgets within a home or office such as computers, TVs, florescent and halogen lights emit electrical fields which can go into the wiring in the walls and cause distortion of the normal electrical waves. Second, whenever electricity leaves a power station, it travels to our homes, offices, and schools through wires, but most of us do not realize that this energy must return to the power station to complete the circuit. Seventy to eighty percent of the returning energy travels through the ground on its way back to the power station. We know that electrical energy takes the path of least resistance, which just might happen to be your home. Electrical fields in the walls of your home may then increase in intensity and also become distorted. Third, high frequency radio waves coming from cellular, broadcast, and other types of communication towers can be a health hazard. The wiring in a building can act like an antenna, picking up these radio waves and thus distorting and boosting the electrical fields in your immediate environment. In summary, these three kinds of extra energy sources can go into the wiring of your home or office, where they emit high intensity energy fields that can have far-reaching effects on cellular function and health.

If a person is exposed to dirty electric fields over a long period of time, a number of symptoms can be associated with what is now called electrical hypersensitivity. These include headaches, dizziness, nausea, difficulty concentrating, memory loss, irritability, depression, anxiety, insomnia, fatigue, weakness, tremors, muscle spasms, numbness, tingling, altered reflexes, muscle and joint pain, seizures, paralysis, and stroke. As well, heart palpitations can occur along with chest pain or pressure, alterations in blood pressure, slow or fast heart rate, shortness of breath, skin rashes, itching, burning sensations, flushing, pain or burning in the eyes, altered vision, floaters, digestive, problems, abdominal pain, enlarged thyroid gland, dryness of the lips, tongue, mouth, and eyes, altered sugar metabolism (diabetes mellitus or low blood sugar), immune system abnormalities, redistribution of metals in the body, hair loss, dental pain, altered sense of smell, and ringing in the ears.[2]

It is easy to identify abnormal, dirty electrical fields by using a relatively inexpensive testing device called the Graham-Stetzer Microsurge Meter, which looks like this:

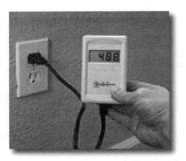

Figure 11.3

When the meter is plugged into an electrical outlet, a digital reading appears within a few seconds. The reading should ideally be 25 or less. If it is much greater than 25, a Graham-Stetzer Filter can be plugged into the outlet, and within a few seconds the digital reading improves dramatically.

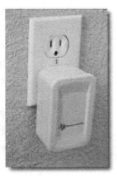

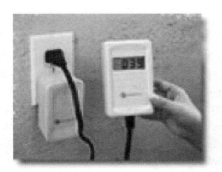

Figure 11.4   Figure 11.5

The entire home should be tested. It can take up to twenty Graham-Stetzer Filters to decrease dirty electric fields sufficiently to improve health. A dramatic improvement in conditions such as multiple sclerosis, diabetes mellitus, autism, and ADHD, among many others, has been documented as a result of using these filters. I encourage you to test your home and office environments and to become informed about the topic of dirty electricity in general.[3]

Galvanic Forces

Galvanic forces are electric fields that are created when dissimilar metals are placed in close proximity. If a solution containing minerals is added, an electric cell is created and the electric current will increase. Mercury amalgams (silver fillings in the teeth) contain five dissimilar metals including mercury, silver, tin, copper, and zinc. The most prevalent metals are mercury (approximately 50 percent) and silver (approximately 35 percent); the remaining amount (15 percent) is made up of the other metals. When these five metals are mixed in an amalgam, an electric current occurs. The strength of the current produced by a typical mercury amalgam is usually between 0.1 and 10 microamps, compared to the body's natural electric current of 3 microamps. Galvanic action increases when other metal alloys such as gold are placed in close proximity to a mercury amalgam. This can also occur if the teeth are apposing or if a gold crown is placed directly over a mercury amalgam.

It is quite common to observe gold crowns sitting across from, or between, mercury amalgams. The biological dentist who works in my clinic often will measure the field strength of amalgams, and he commonly observes large amounts of electric current. One main issue is that electric currents in the mouth will draw out mercury, as well as the other metals in amalgams, at a higher rate. These metals can then be breathed in, or they can be driven into the surrounding tissues, and it is important to remember that the brain is very close by.

One man whom I had treated for iron overload told me that from the time he was young he would hear a radio station in his head, but when his mercury amalgams were removed, the radio stopped playing. He could hear the radio because the mercury amalgams in his mouth operated as an antenna for radio signals. Often patients tell me that when they get their last amalgams removed, they experience sudden clarity of mind, reduction of headaches, resolution of tinnitus, improved vision and sinuses, and many other, more subtle, symptoms.

Scars

Another, less well-known source of galvanic action in our bodies is scars, as physicians in Europe have recognized for the past eighty years. Any scar resulting from an accident, a surgical procedure, or an illness can produce long-lasting effects on a person's health.

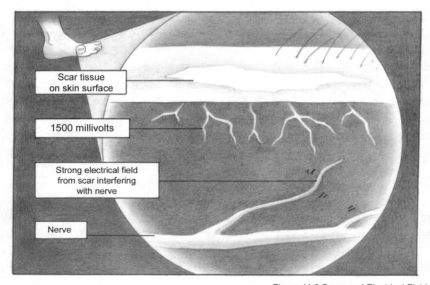

Scar tissue on skin surface

1500 millivolts

Strong electrical field from scar interfering with nerve

Nerve

Figure 11.6 Scars and Electrical Fields

Scars and other sites of physical trauma in the body can generate electrical fields producing a measurable electrical charge of up to 1.5 V (1500 millivolts). This is about nineteen times greater than the normal resting cell membrane potential (80 millivolts). In turn, the electrical field created by scar tissue can interfere with the nervous system, much like a battery inappropriately implanted in the body. Electrical chaos might then occur in the spinal cord and brain, producing a cascade of nerve disturbances throughout the body, which may manifest as chronic pain or organ dysfunction.

By simply injecting a local anesthetic into a scar, we can create a nerve block that allows the millions of nerves in the scar to restore their normal resting membrane potential. The local effect of the anesthetic usually lasts between two and three hours, which is enough time for the cell to eliminate toxic waste products. Sometimes, this is the only therapeutic intervention necessary, but often other toxic factors are present that also require intervention.

The usual treatment course for scars is five weekly injections using preservative-free 0.5 percent or 1.0 percent procaine. Other effective methods include the use of laser or pulsating electric fields. Let me now introduce you to Susan, whose case provides a compelling example of how effective the treatment of scars can be.

Susan's Case

In 1999, Susan, a sixty-one-year-old woman with a master's degree in social work, came to my clinic complaining of chronic lower back pain, which she began to experience after a car accident thirty years earlier. The pain gradually became generalized, and eventually she was diagnosed with fibromyalgia. For years she also had suffered with recurrent migraine headaches. When I met her, she was on several medications, including 20 mg daily of

Paxil® (an antidepressant), 7.5 mg daily of Imovane® (a sedative), and four Percocet® (a strong synthetic narcotic combined with acetaminophen) per day. Ten years before she attended my clinic, she had to give up her job in social work administration because of her chronic pain.

As I took her history, I discovered that Susan had undergone a large number of surgical procedures, including tonsillectomy as child, uterine suspension/appendectomy, hysterectomy, right breast biopsy, fusion of vertebrae C 1 - 3, bilateral bunionectomy, wisdom teeth extraction, laparoscopy, right elbow extensor tendon release, arthroscopy (right knee), rhinoplasty (nose surgery), lumbar decompression and laminectomy, and fusion of her right first toe. Susan brought with her a thick folder filled with a myriad of laboratory investigations, all of which were within normal limits. She had suffered for years and continued to be in severe and constant pain. Given her history, it is not surprising that Susan had a multitude of scars on her body. She had no mercury amalgams present, she had difficulty walking heel-to-toe, all fibromyalgia tender points tested positive, and she had decreased motion of the cervical and lumbar spines.

I decided to begin by injecting her scars with one percent preservative-free procaine, and, remarkably, within one hour of treatment she went for a walk and realized that she was able to climb stairs without pain. Soon after, she discovered that her generalized pain had decreased significantly, and for the first time in years she did not take her narcotic painkillers and slept well. She also observed that her balance had improved significantly. Four days later, before she returned to Toronto, Ontario, her scars were reinjected, and she was referred to a physician in Toronto who does similar work. She experienced what is known as the "lightning phenomenon" – a sudden resolution of symptoms within a short time after treatment. A DMPS challenge test was also done, and revealed a moderate amount of mercury, lead, and tin being excreted in her urine.

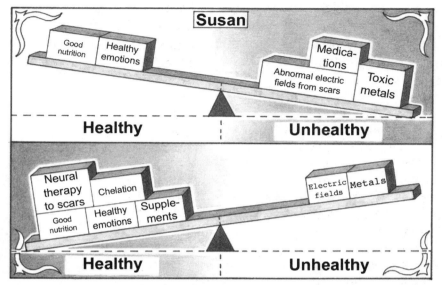

Figure 11.7 Susan

Summary

Injecting scars with a local anesthetic is one of several treatment modalities used in a discipline called neural therapy, which originated in Germany in the 1920s and is practiced by a large number of European physicians. A growing number of physicians in North America have also taken the training and have achieved highly significant results.[4]

It has been my clinical experience that most people with electromagnetic sensitivity are generally very toxic with metals, persistent organic pollutants, and mycotoxins, and often they have toxic teeth or jawbones. Although neural therapy alone is not sufficient to treat such a range of problems, it can be an effective

153

component in a treatment program. Europe is far ahead of North America in the study of electromagnetic sensitivity, but interest in this topic is growing throughout the world, and new information is rapidly being made available.

---

[1] Li DK, et al. 2002. A population-based prospective cohort study of personal exposure to magnetic fields during pregnancy and the risk of miscarriage. Epidemiology. 13: 9 - 20.

[2] Havas M. Electromagnetic hypersensitivity: biological effects of dirty electricity with emphasis on diabetes and multiple sclerosis. Electromagn Biol Med. 2006;25(4):259-68. Review.

[3] More information on dirty electricity can be found at www.dirtyelectricity.ca

[4] www.neuraltherapy.com

Our Toxic Mouths

There are four main ways our mouths can be the source of increased toxic load on the body: first, the release of mercury from dental amalgams; second, the galvanic (electric) effect from having dissimilar metals in close proximity, thereby creating abnormally high electrical fields near the brain; third, infections associated with the teeth, causing a release of toxins into the system; and fourth, osteonecrosis (bone death) of the jawbones. We have already dealt with the harmful effects of mercury and electromagnetic fields, and in this chapter I want to focus on the important topic of osteonecrosis. But first, a few words about oral infections.

Oral Infections

There is a strong connection between oral toxicity and systemic disease, and over the past decade a wealth of published research confirms this point. An unhealthy mouth can lead to such things as heart attack, stroke, high blood pressure, atherosclerosis (hardening of the arteries), infections of artificial joints, various forms of arthritis, systemic infection, brain abscesses, cancer, and preterm and low birth weight babies.[1]

Studies have shown also that microorganisms, including bacteria and yeast from teeth-related infections, can spread throughout the body and in favorable conditions these organisms can reestablish themselves in other organs, thereby causing disease. Furthermore, if there is infection around a tooth (periodontal disease), the harmful organisms can move into the tooth,[2] and if the tooth is dead because of a root canal procedure, the organisms can take up residence in the millions of little tubules inside the tooth.

These organisms can then spread, resulting in endodontic disease, which destroys the bone (osteonecrosis).[3] To make matters worse, anaerobic bacteria (bacteria that do not require oxygen in order to thrive) can feed on the tissue surrounding the infection and produce families of toxins known as exotoxins. Examples of exotoxins include hydrogen sulfide gas, putrescene (diaminobutane), and cadaverine (diaminopentanein). Each of these exotoxins inhibits a number of key enzymes that are necessary for energy production,[4] while also adversely affecting protein synthesis and stimulating overproduction of proinflammatory cells. Unpublished research indicates that exotoxins can inhibit gene expression, thereby causing cancer.[5] The amount of enzyme inhibition caused by exotoxins can now be quantified by a technique called "affinity labeling analysis," developed by Boyd Haley, PhD, and his researchers at the University of Kentucky.[6]

Osteonecrosis

The term osteonecrosis means "bone that is dead."[7] Of all the bones in the body, the jawbones (upper maxilla and lower mandible) suffer the most consistent trauma, caused by the everyday activity of chewing food and by dental procedures. For instance, when wisdom teeth are extracted, in the large majority of cases a chronic, silent bone infection occurs which can be present for decades with few, if any, local symptoms.[8] Other causes of osteonecrosis are trauma, use of adrenaline in local anesthetics, radiation therapy, infection and inflammation from teeth, failed root canal therapy, overheating of bone during surgery or dental procedures, corticosteroid injection of bone, elevated blood pressure in the bone, and trauma from occlusion. Osteonecrosis can also occur as a result of corticosteroid therapy (using prednisone or prednisolone), biphosphonate drugs for treating osteoporosis, atmospheric pressure changes in certain occupations (for instance, deep-sea diving), blood clotting disorders, estrogen therapy, pregnancy, alcohol abuse, cancer chemotherapy, sickle cell anemia, systemic lupus erythematosus, homocystinemia, osteoporosis, hyperlipidemia, and smoking.

Recently published research shows that the majority of people with osteonecrosis, whether in the jawbone or elsewhere, have minor defects in their ability to coagulate, making them more prone to develop micro-clots in the tiny arterioles supplying the bone.[9] Because these micro-clots prevent blood from nourishing the bone, osteonecrosis occurs more easily. If an osteonecrotic lesion begins in the jawbone, it gradually expands through the porous alveolar bone that makes up the central part of the jawbone; this looks somewhat like sponge-toffee. See Figure 12.1.[10]

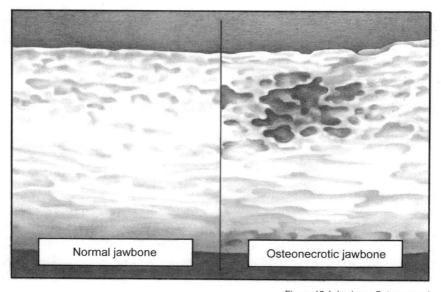

Normal jawbone

Osteonecrotic jawbone

Figure 12.1 Jawbone Osteonecrosis

When a jawbone lesion reaches the mandibular branch of the facial nerve, severe pain can result.[11] The term for this condition is Neuralgia Inducing Cavitational Osteonecrosis (NICO). Interestingly, Dr. G. V. Black (the father of modern dentistry) described these lesions as early as 1915; he devoted an entire section of his classic textbook, *A Work on Special Dental Pathology,* to this subject.

Over sixty disease processes are known to be associated with osteonecrotic lesions, including hypercoagulation states (conditions causing blood to clot excessively) and cancer. Until recently, these lesions were almost impossible to diagnose without surgery because there has been no reliable way to test for them by using x-rays. Fortunately, a new technology using Through-Transmission Alveolar Ultrasonography (TAU) has been developed and approved by the FDA in the U.S. and the Health Protection Branch in Canada.[12] This unit is known as Cavitat 4000, and it has a 98 percent sensitivity – which means that 98 percent of the time if there is an osteonecrotic lesion present, this technology will pick it up.

Lori's Case

Lori was a forty-nine-year-old self-employed businesswoman who had a four-year history of severe left mandibular (lower jawbone) pain. Her symptoms began when she suddenly developed pain in the first molar left mandible. Fourteen years before the pain developed, she had a gold crown placed in that location. She also had her wisdom teeth extracted.

Loris's pain gradually became worse, and her dentist treated her by performing a root canal on the painful tooth. She was then referred to an endodontist, and as a result she had two gold crowns with root canals placed in the upper left molars. Unfortunately, the pain in the left lateral mandibular region became worse, and Lori was referred to a prosthodontist, who fashioned a splint that made no difference whatsoever to her pain. She was then referred to an ear, nose, and throat specialist, who suggested that she had isolated dental pain with possible nerve inflammation. An oral surgeon found that the crown associated with the pain appeared to be satisfactory, and an x-ray of the left mandible revealed a normal-appearing jawbone with possible scar tissue at the root tip of the tooth in question. The oral surgeon then performed a series of nerve blocks, but these still did not have any effect on Loris's chronic pain. She finally consulted a neurologist, and was placed on a series of medications, including an anticonvulsant and an antidepressant. The antidepressant gave some relief from the pain, but Lori gained thirty-five pounds and was able to work only part-time. Seven months before she came to my clinic, she discontinued the antidepressant, and the pain escalated to a point where she became suicidal.

When I examined her, Lori appeared tired, worn-out, and she wept easily. Her fingernails showed signs that she had zinc deficiency, and her balance testing was abnormal. She had thirteen mercury amalgams, as well as three gold crowns. The lateral portion of her left lower jaw was very tender to touch. I told her that she probably was suffering from NICO (Neuralgia Inducing Cavitational Osteonecrosis), and if that were the case, we should be able to assist her. She promptly burst into tears.

We performed a Cavitat scan, which revealed presumptive evidence of osteonecrosis under Lori's molars on the lateral side of her left lower jawbone. (see Figure 12.2)

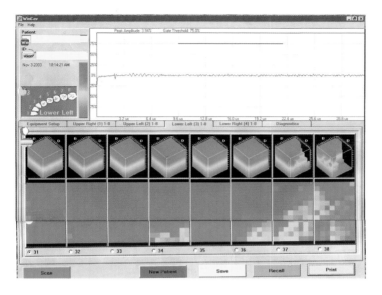

Figure 12.2 Cavitat #1 Pretreatment

Cavitat #1 Pretreatment

The normal images on the left side of the scan show solid three-dimensional blocks representing normal bone. In the two-dimensional images underneath, normal bone is represented by solid green rectangles. Yellow represents inflamed bone, orange represents necrotic (dead) bone, and red represents an empty space where there is no bone at all. Lori's first Cavitat scan shows presumptive evidence of absent and necrotic bone just underneath the place where the wisdom tooth used to be. The bone under the root-canal-treated tooth is two squares to the left, and the scan shows presumptive evidence of inflamed, necrotic bone at that site.

With this evidence in hand, I referred Lori to a dentist skilled in dealing with NICO lesions. The dentist initially performed a series of local anesthetic injections into Lori's jawbone near the affected site, and within ten minutes her pain had completely resolved, which confirmed the working diagnosis of NICO. The dentist then performed limited surgery to her jawbone, opening up the region of decayed bone and removing as much as he could. A specimen was sent for analysis, and Lori was given a device containing high intensity red and infrared light emitting diodes (LEDs) that she applied to her cheek for fifteen minutes each day. She used this device for three months.

Two weeks after Lori's first dental procedure, she had complete resolution of the severe pain that had plagued her for four years, and she was able to discontinue her pain and antidepressant medications. The pathology report showed that she indeed had necrosis at the tip of the root canal. During the following months, a series of Cavitat scans showed complete restoration of new bone in the lateral left lower jawbone. (see Figures 12.3 - 12.6)

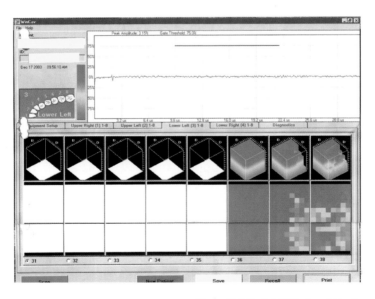

Figure 12.3 Cavitat #2 Post-op 1 Month

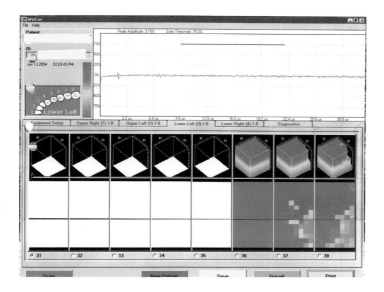

Figure 12.4 Cavitat #3 Post-op 2 Months

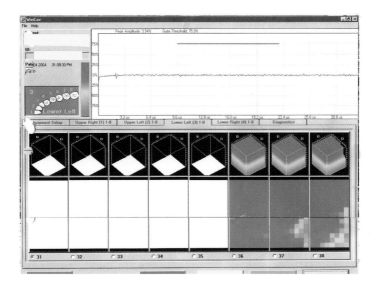

Figure 12.5 Cavitat #4 Post-op 4 Months

163

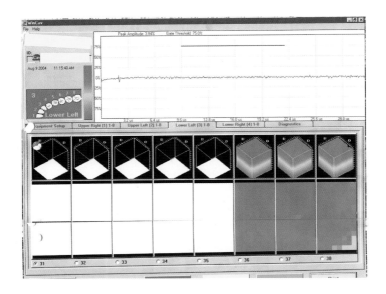

Figure 12.6 Cavitat #5 Post-op 10 Months

Case Discussion

This is an excellent case for demonstrating how an osteonecrotic lesion can cause severe pain if it affects the mandibular nerve. In Lori's case, the pain was so unbearable and persistent that she contemplated suicide. Using the TILT Phenomenon, we can see how a number of factors contributed to Lori's loss of health.

Her wisdom teeth extractions could have caused the osteonecrosis process to begin. Fourteen years before the onset of pain she had a gold crown placed above the roots of the problem molar, thereby causing trauma to the tooth. The root canal placed in the problem molar was eventually found to have a necrotic tip. Lori had thirteen mercury amalgams that were constantly releasing mercury and having an impact on her general immune system function, while adding to her toxic load. Taken together, these factors caused the right side of the balance to tilt downwards, but

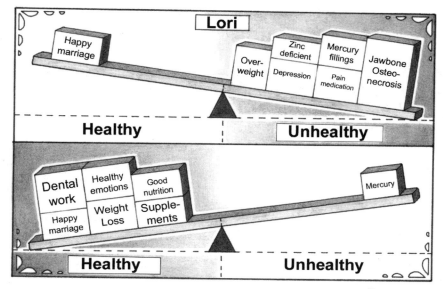

Figure 12.7 Lori

every attempt to shift the balance back to normal was ineffective until the underlying necrosis was diagnosed. Proper treatment resulted in removal of the toxic focus in her body, following which she experienced a rapid shift of her health back towards normal. The next step in her recovery will be careful removal of the mercury amalgams in her teeth in conjunction with a detoxification program. To confirm how devastating the effects of osteonecrosis are, I would like to consider one more case.

Richard's Case

Richard was sixty-two years old when he came to me for an allergy consultation. He was taking prednisone (a powerful steroid), and I assumed this was to treat his severe allergic rhinitis (hay fever), but Richard explained that he was taking prednisone for a severe and chronically painful condition in his muscles that he had experienced over the previous three years. It soon became apparent to me that he was suffering with polymyalgia rheumatica, a severe inflammatory condition of the muscles, the cause of which is unknown. If the diagnosis is missed and treatment with steroid drugs is not implemented, irreversible blindness can develop. For the first year and a half Richard had used prednisone daily, shifting thereafter to shorter courses on a monthly basis. He told me that he did not like taking this powerful drug, but his doctor had told him there was no other treatment available.

When I asked Richard the key question about whether or not he had undergone dental work, he stated that he had a root canal performed on one of his left lower molars six months prior to onset of his severe muscle pain. When he developed extreme pain in the left lower jaw laterally, he ordered his dentist to remove the tooth with the root canal, but the pain persisted and gradually became worse. Taking prednisone did not help, and Richard supplemented it with over-the-counter pain medications.

Richard's other medical conditions included osteoarthritis and high cholesterol, for which he was not on medication. He appeared older than his actual age, and his blood pressure was somewhat elevated. He had tenderness along his left lower mandible, as well as in the associated glands in his upper left region of his neck. The membranes in his nasal passages were chronically swollen, and his knees showed signs of chronic osteoarthritis.

Richard's multiple investigations were normal except for an elevated sedimentation rate (this is a blood test for the presence of inflammation in the body). The test result was 24 mm/hr (with normal being 0-20). His cholesterol and triglycerides were somewhat elevated, and his chest x-ray was normal. An x-ray of his jawbone revealed an absence of all molars in the lower left jaw and no signs of bone necrosis. Richard attended my clinic one month before we received our Cavitat 4000 ultrasound unit, so we were not able to perform a Cavitat scan on him, but I told Richard that he was probably suffering from NICO, and I referred him to a dentist skilled in dealing with these lesions.

The dentist opened up Richard's left lower lateral jawbone region. He discovered a large, cavernous lesion that extended back towards the angle of the jaw and up towards the ear. He removed as much necrotic bone as possible, and, within a few days, the chronic pain in Richard's lower left jawbone disappeared, and his energy and sense of well-being began to increase. The swollen glands in his upper left neck region also returned to normal, and, more importantly, the chronic pain in his muscles disappeared, and he has never had to take prednisone again. He resumed golfing and has pursued his retirement with great enthusiasm.

Case Discussion

Richard had previous extractions of two of the three molars in his left lower jaw. These extractions could have initiated a smoldering osteonecrosis in that region, which might help to explain why he developed pain in the remaining molar resulting in a root canal procedure – yet Richard's pain intensified in spite of having that last molar extracted. At the time of the dental surgery I recommended, it became obvious that he had a large, cavernous osteonecrotic lesion present. A constant stream of exotoxins had been going into his system for several years, so the balance eventually tipped and his health deteriorated. Taking a careful history, recognizing the underlying diagnosis, and removing the toxic focus resulted in a rapid improvement in Richard's health.

Does this mean that all cases of polymyalgia rheumatica are caused by osteonecrosis? I doubt that this is the case, even though recently published research indicates that quite a number of rheumatic conditions indeed are associated with osteonecrosis.[13] Polymyalgia rheumatica is a true inflammatory disorder; for some reason, unknown triggers stimulate the immune system, and the muscles become extremely painful. It is not clear how this happens, and further research is necessary.

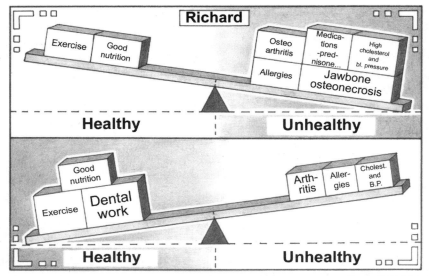

Figure 12.8 Richard

In my clinical practice I have found that toxicity originating in the mouth is often the key to making an effective diagnosis of a whole range of disorders. A few years ago, I attended a conference in Phoenix, Arizona, where I happened to sit next to a physician from Spain. When he heard that I had taken training in neural therapy, he told me that in his many years of clinical practice he estimated that more than 90 per cent of diseases originate from the "neck upwards." I am finding this to be true, and I hope that you will remember to think about the various ways that toxicity originating in your mouth may be a key factor in explaining why you are not as healthy as you feel you should be.

Our Toxic Mouths

[1] Slavkin and Baum. Relationship of dental and oral pathology to systemic illness. JAMA 2000, 284:1215-1217.

Espinola-Klein C, et al. Impact of Infectious Burden on Extent and Long-Term Prognosis of Atherosclerosis. Circulation 2002 Jan 1; 105(1): 15-21.

Loesche. Association of the oral flora with important medical diseases. Curr. Opin. Periodontol. 1997, 4:21-28.

Michaud DS, Joshipura K, Giovannucci E, Fuchs CS. A prospective study of periodontal disease and pancreatic cancer in US male health professionals. J Natl Cancer Inst. 2007 Jan 17; 99(2):171-5.

[2] Debelian et al. Anaerobic bacteremia and fungemia in patients undergoing endodontic therapy: an overview. Ann. Periodontol. 1998; 3:281-287.

Debelian et al. Observation of Saccharomyces cerevisiae in blood of patient undergoing root canal treatment. Int. Endod. J. 1997; 30:313-317.

Debelian et al. Bacteremia in conjunction with endodontic therapy. Endod. Dent. Traumatol. 1995; 11:142-149.

Debelian et al., Systemic diseases caused by oral microorganisms. Endod. Dent. Traumatol. 1994; 10:57-65.

Adriaens et al. Ultrastructural observations on bacterial invasion in cementum and radicular dentin of periodontally diseased human teeth. J. Periodontol. 1998; 59:493-503.

[3] Nagaoka et al. Bacterial invasion into dentinal tubules of human vital and nonvital teeth. J. Endod. 1995; 21:70-73.

Ando and Hishino. Predominant obligate anaerobes invading the deep layers of root canal dentin. Int. Endod. 1990; J. 23:20-27.

[4] Geerts SO, et al. Systemic Release of Endotoxins Induced by Gentle Mastication: Association With Periodontitis Severity. J Periodontol 2002 Jan; 73(1): 73-8.

Langendijk PS, Hanssen JT, Van der Hoeven JS. Sulfate-reducing bacteria in association with human periodontitis. J. Clin Periodontol. 2000 Dec 27; (12): 943-50.

Persson et al. The formation of hydrogen sulfide and methyl mercaptan by oral bacteria. Oral Microbiol. Immunol. 1990; 5:195-201.

Waler. On the transformation of sulfur-containing amino acids and peptides to volatile sulfur compounds (VSC) in the human mouth. Eur. J. Oral Sci. 1997; 105:534-537.

Lamster et al. The polyamines putrescine, spermidine and spermine in human gingival crevicular fluid. Arch. Oral Biol. 1987; 32:329-333.

Masui and Kirimura. Production of putrescine from arginine by oral microorganisms. Shigaku. 1987; 75:117-136.

Maita and Horiuchi. Polyamine analysis of infected root canal contents related to clinical symptoms. Endod. Dent. Traumatol. 1990; 6:213-217.

Finkelstein and Benevenga. The effect of methanethiol and methionine toxicity on the activities of cytochrome c oxidase and enzymes involved in protection from peroxidative damage. J. Nutr. 1986; 116:204-2.

[5] Jones B, et al. 2003. P53 and its associates P21, CDK2 and Cancer. Lecture 3rd Cavitat Workshop and Educational Conference Jan 17-18 Denver CO. www.cavitat.com.

[6] Perdergrass, J.C. 2001. Toxins Produced by Oral Microorganisms: Adverse Effects On Vital Body Enzymes and Detection in Oral Samples. Lecture presented at the Third Annual Dental, Medical, and Scientific Conference on Sources, Diagnosis and Treatment of Oral Toxicities May 2001. University of Kentucky.

[7] Soucacos PN. Osteonecrosis of the human skeleton. Orthop Clin North Am. 2004; 35(3): xiii-xv

[8] Shankland WE II. 2002. Medullary and Odontogenic Disease in the Painful Jaw: Clinicopathologic Review of 500 Consecutive Lesions. J Craniomandib Prac. Vol 20 No.4. 295-303.

[9] Korompilias AV. Coagulation abnormalities in patients with hip osteonecrosis. Orthop Clin North Am. 2004; 35(3): 265-71, vii.

[10] Adams WR, et al. J Oral Pathol Med 1999; 28:423.

[11] Bouquot JE, McMahon RE. Neuropathic pain in maxillofacial osteonecrosis. J Oral Maxillofac Surg. 2000 Sep; 58(9): 1003-20. Review.

[12] Bouquot JE, et al. Through-transmission Alveolar Ultrasonography (TAU) – new technology for evaluation of bone density and desiccation. Comparison with radiology of 170 biopsied alveolar sites of osteoporotic and ischemic disease. Oral Surg Oral Med Oral Pathol Oral Radiol Endod. 2002; 93:214-215.

Bouquot JE, et al. Through-transmission Alveolar Ultrasonography (TAU) – new technology for detection of low bone density of the jaws. Comparison with radiology for 92 osteoporotic alveolar sites with histopathologic confirmation. J Oral Pathol Med. 2002; 31:289-290.

Shankland WE, Bouquot JE. Focal osteoporotic marrow defect: report of 100 new cases with ultrasonography scans. Cranio. 2004 Oct; 22(4):314-9.

[13] Tektonidou MG. Immunologic factors in the pathogenesis of osteonecrosis. Orthop Clin North Am - 01-JUL-2004; 35(3): 259-63, vii

Water - Damage at the Source

Besides air, water is the most basic sustaining substance we put into our bodies. Alarmingly, many people spend thousands of dollars on supplements, gym memberships, organic foods, and so on, but neglect to drink high-quality water in adequate amounts. Yet simply drinking enough high-quality water each day can produce many health benefits, such as improved digestion and absorption of nutrients into the cells; a decreased incidence of kidney stones, urinary tract infections, and constipation; an accelerated excretion of toxins and waste products from the body through the urine, feces, breath, and sweat; weight loss and weight control by decreased cravings for sugars; lubrication of joints and muscles, resulting in reduced inflammation and accelerated healing when injuries occur; a boost in cognitive function (as little as 2 percent dehydration can decrease short-term memory, as is commonly seen in elderly people). By contrast, an insufficient intake of high-quality water can result in a worsening of many chronic health conditions, such as arthritis, muscle pain, high blood pressure, asthma, and headaches.

Our Toxic Water

Most tap water has been processed through treatment plants, and although a large number of impurities are removed, substances such as chlorine and aluminum sulfate are added into the water, and these can be harmful to our health. The Environmental Protection Agency (EPA) has reported that individuals who drink and bathe in municipal treated (chlorinated) water obtained from lakes, rivers, or shallow wells, have a higher chance of developing cancer.[2] Municipal water is often found to contain traces of organic chemicals such as pesticides, MTBE (a gasoline additive), heavy metals, parasites, and radioactive compounds. If we drink and bathe in this type of water, levels of these harmful compounds will gradually increase in our bodies. Furthermore, most of us do not realize that a ten-minute shower can result in a 600 percent increase in absorption of contaminants, as compared to the contaminants in water consumed orally in one day. It is therefore of the highest importance to consume high-quality water as part of a detoxification and health restoration program.

Prior to becoming one of my patients, a woman who realized the importance of proper hydration began to consume larger amounts of water throughout the day, but, perplexingly, felt worse as a result. At first, she thought that feeling worse might be part of her health restoration, a "detoxification effect," and so she consumed even more water. She then noticed that her energy was seriously depleted, and her memory was not what it should be. She also developed muscle pains and became depressed. Her doctor placed her on an antidepressant medication, but her health continued to deteriorate. Finally, she saw a naturopathic physician who performed a hair analysis, which revealed high levels of copper. It was soon discovered that her tap water also had excessively high levels of copper. Further investigation revealed that the water from the well on her property was acidic, and the water pipes in her house were made of copper. One result of acidic water sitting in copper pipes is that copper is leached out. The naturopath first made sure that the patient switched to good quality drinking water, and then treated her with a high intake of zinc, as well as an oral chelating agent. As a result of these treatments, her symptoms cleared up.

Contaminated water can indeed play havoc with our health, but my patient was also correct in the first place to think that drinking excellent water is of the highest importance if detoxification is to occur effectively. Today, many water purification systems are readily available, and there are a multitude of claims as to which is the best. Some of my patients use distilled water, but this type of water is quite acidic. Other patients have had reverse osmosis units installed in their homes (as I did), but a great deal of water is required for this process, and the water produced is devoid of minerals. Some of my patients ozonate their water, and also run it in front of ultraviolet lights to kill any microorganisms that may be present.

The best water purification system that I have come across, which I now use both at home and in my clinic, is the Wellness Filter®. This is a Japanese product, and research confirms that it is highly effective. It is easy to install, simple to use, and relatively inexpensive. As tap water percolates through the various layers, contaminants are removed and minerals are added. A final step involves passing the decontaminated and mineralized water through magnetic fields that reorganize the water molecules into clusters.

I recommend the Wellness Filter® based on personal experience. (I do not own any shares in the company, and I do not profit from any sales or promotion of these units). My main concern is simply to emphasize the importance of drinking plentiful amounts of high quality water. After all, the blood running through our arteries and veins is approximately 90 percent water, which means that water is constantly moving through our bodies and transporting goods and waste products as our blood supplies various nutrients and gets rid of toxic waste products. It takes approximately twelve minutes for water in the blood to circulate completely through our bodies, and each day our livers filter approximately 200 liters of blood. In short, the inner workings of our bodies depend greatly on water, which explains why the average human is composed of approximately 70 percent water, of which approximately 75 percent is stored within our cells. However, as we progress through life, the amount of water in our bodies gradually decreases. When we are in our mother's womb, we are approximately 99 percent water, but in infancy this percentage drops to 90, and by the time we have reached adulthood, our water content drops to approximately 70 percent. In our elderly years, the amount of water in our bodies diminishes even further, to about 50 percent.

It is all too easy to ignore how dehydration can affect our general health, and we are well advised to make a conscious effort to ensure that we are adequately hydrated. Authorities on this topic suggest that each of us should drink half of our body weight in ounces of water each day, which for a 150-pound person would be 75 ounces. We should remember that the water circulating inside us, giving us life, is the same water that circulates through our environment; there is a constant motion and circulation of life-giving water everywhere on the planet, as the simple illustration below indicates.

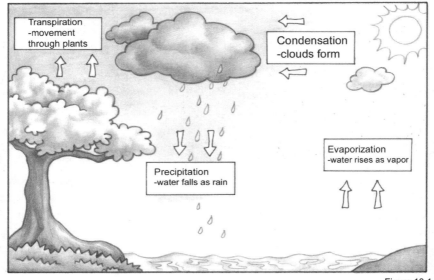

Figure 13.1

Water, then, is as essential to the composition of our bodies as it is to life itself, and the wonders and mysteries of water always give me pleasure to contemplate. My family and I are very fortunate to be able to live right next to the Strait of Georgia on the east side of beautiful Vancouver Island in British Columbia, Canada. Almost every day, I walk to the beach so that I can see and hear the waves as they come crashing onto the shore. I love the salty smell of the ocean, the harbor seals, the occasional killer whale, and the various birds, including bald eagles. I also enjoy walking in the rain (as long as it is not too cold), and swimming gives me a sense of freedom and exhilaration.

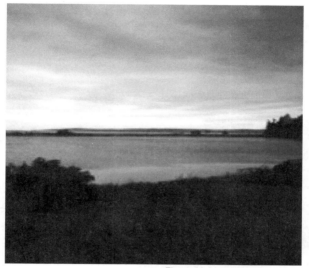

Figure 13.2 View from My House

The wonders and life-giving power of water are, for me, unfailingly interesting to contemplate, while also serving as a reminder of how important it is to make sure that our bodies are plentifully supplied with this remarkable substance, so basic to life itself. With the wonders of water in mind, I will end this chapter by citing the work of Dr. Masuru Emoto[1], a Japanese doctor of alternative medicine whose main interest has been to explore the mysteries of water. Among other things, Dr. Emoto provides remarkable pictures of water crystals, about which he makes highly interesting observations.

If water is frozen and then brought back to the point of thaw, crystals form on the surface and can be studied under a microscope. Dr. Emoto claims that these crystals change shape in ways that reflect such influences as the emotions of the observer, words spoken, and the quality of sounds in the near vicinity. He also claims that the crystal structure of water can change for better or for worse. For instance, praying over water will actually improve its crystal structure, and the most beautiful crystal formations apparently occur when the observer expresses love and gratitude. The following pictures are taken by Dr. Emoto and are available on the Internet.

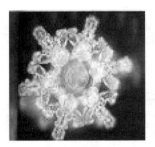

Figure 13.3 Pure Water

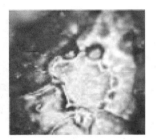

Figure 13.4 Polluted Water

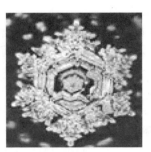

Figure 13.5 Polluted Water after Prayer

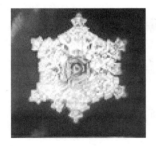

Figure 13.6 Classical Music

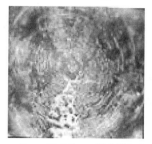

Figure 13.7 Heavy Metal Music

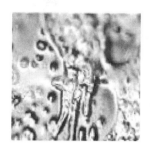

Figure 13.8 "I Hate You"

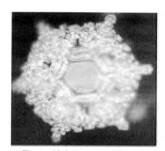

Figure 13.9 "Love and Gratitude"

Although there is much work yet to be done on this topic, Dr. Emoto's experiments remind us again of the importance of pure water – which, like our cells, is delicate, amazingly complex, and easily ruined by pollution. Dr. Emoto's experiments also suggest that our physical health is not just something that can be measured objectively, but includes our emotions. As his experiments suggest, there is no clear boundary between the objective and subjective worlds, and this leads me to my next chapter, on the danger of toxic emotions.

[1] Emoto M. *The Hidden Messages in Water*. Hillsboro, Oregon: Beyond Words Publishing; 2004.

[2] Wilkins JR 3rd, et.al. <http://www.ncbi.nlm.nih.gov/pubmed/389042?ordinalpos=49&itool=EntrezSystem2.PEntrez.Pubmed.Pubmed_ResultsPanel.Pubmed_RVDocSum> Organic chemical contaminants in drinking water and cancer. Am J Epidemiol. 1979 Oct;110(4):420-48. Review

Toxic Emotions

The importance of emotional health is not often discussed when a physician treats people suffering with chronic illnesses such as cancer, heart disease, diabetes mellitus, or autoimmune diseases such as rheumatoid arthritis or lupus. Over the past several decades, the emphasis on biochemistry, the pharmaceutical industry, and "a drug for every bug" has promoted a widespread idea that illness can be cured by instrumental means in much the same way as we might repair a broken-down car. Still, a wide range of health practitioners, including psychiatrists, psychologists, counselors, and medical doctors know very well that our emotions affect our health directly, and, as Dr. Emoto's experiments with water crystals suggest, there is no clear line between the external world and our interior, subjective experience.

Although in this book I have so far been dealing mostly with the effects on our health of toxic substances in the environment outside us, it is appropriate now to mention briefly the ill effects of toxic emotions and the significance of acquiring "emotional competence." To explain what I mean by emotional competence, let me return briefly to the seesaw model which I used to introduce the idea of the TILT Phenomenon. In our emotional lives, stress also can build to a tipping point in much the same way our bodies respond to the physical effects of toxins. Emotional competence consists of strategies and techniques that we can use to counteract the stresses which build over time until our emotional stability tilts and we become ill.

Stress and Modern Living

Dr. Hans Selye, a distinguished neurologist who coined the term "stress response," points out that "stress is not simply nervous tension," but also a measurable set of physiological events in the body.[1] And in his impressive book, *When the Body Says No: The Cost of Hidden Stress,* Gabor Mate argues that chronically repressed negative emotions (especially anger) contribute significantly to physical disease in our highly stressed-out world.[2] As both of these highly capable authorities suggest, our emotions affect our physical health, and Dr. Selye has compiled a list of danger signals that can alert us to the fact that we are experiencing undue stress.[3] These include such physical symptoms as a pounding or racing heart, chest pain, lightheadedness, shortness of breath, sweating, dry mouth, constipation, diarrhea, upset stomach, frequent urination, tremor, headaches, muscle aches, stiffness of the neck or jaws, weight gain or weight loss, high blood pressure, sexual problems, and fatigue. Emotional states such as anxiety, loss of the joy of life, over-alertness, and tension also provide warnings, as do behavioral traits such as impulsivity, irritability, insomnia, or exaggerated reactions to events.

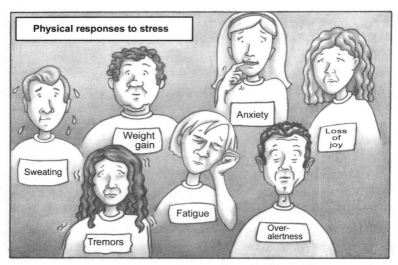

Figure 14.1 Physical Responses to Stress

Many of us are chronically overstressed today because the primitive emotions of fear and aggression are kept active by the competitiveness and anxieties of modern living. That is, we live continuously in conditions that alarm us in much the same way as our remote ancestors were alarmed by meeting predatory animals. In such a situation, the brain sends out signals through the nervous system, and stress hormones such as adrenaline and cortisol are released very quickly, preparing us for "fight or flight." Signals are also sent to the immune system, which ramps up its production of various cells, such as the natural killer cells that are designed to protect us in the event of an attack. Clearly, it is not good for us to live in conditions which cause a constant release of stress hormones, but that is what too many of us find ourselves doing in the modern world.

The Steps to Emotional Competence

In the first few years of life, our nervous, hormonal, and immune systems mature. If we are raised in a loving and nurturing home, we will learn to express our emotions appropriately. However, no home is perfect and there are no perfect parents; consequently, all of us are to some degree emotionally traumatized when we are very young. Some of us are more seriously traumatized than others, and serious trauma leads to the mal-expression of emotions and to their unhealthy repression. Mate points out that the repression of negative emotions such as anger drives our nervous, hormonal, and immune systems into chronic states of stress that can remain hidden from our minds for decades until we reach a tipping point, with disastrous consequences for our health.

One goal for each of us is therefore to develop a balanced emotional life, sometimes referred to as "emotional competence." As Mate says, "emotional competence is the capacity that enables us to stand in a responsible, non-victimized, and non-self-harming relationship with our environment. It is the required internal ground for facing life's inevitable stresses, for avoiding the creation of unnecessary ones, and for furthering the healing process. Few of us reach adult age with anything close to full emotional competence."[4] In short, just as our physical environment today is polluted, so also is our subjective environment, and these two conditions mirror one another. Nonetheless, we should seek physical health as much as possible, and likewise we should attempt to achieve emotional competence.

Four basic criteria define what emotional competence is, and Mate also provides a list of seven steps that can assist us in achieving it. The four criteria are as follows: (1) a capacity to feel our emotions, so that we are aware when we are experiencing stress; (2) an ability to express our emotions effectively, thereby asserting our needs and maintaining the integrity of our emotional boundaries; (3) an ability to distinguish between psychological reactions that are pertinent to the present situation and those that represent a residue from the past. (That is, the demands we make upon the world should conform to our present needs and not to unconscious, unsatisfied needs from childhood. If the distinctions between past and present are blurred, we can all too readily perceive loss, or the threat of loss, where none exists); (4) an awareness of genuine needs that require satisfaction rather than repression for the sake of gaining the acceptance or approval others.

To enable us to achieve these goals, Mate lists the following seven steps:[5]

1.) Acceptance. This implies that we are willing to accept life as it is and open ourselves to a realistic appraisal of our situation. Frequently, we are more accommodating and less judgmental of others than of ourselves, and we correct this imbalance by being more compassionate towards ourselves.

2.) Awareness. In our fast-paced world it is often difficult to be aware of our changing emotional states and their significance. Yet, we must be able to recognize emotions that accompany our experiences of stress. Careful attention can assist us to do this and to avoid the unhealthy suppression of emotions that should be acknowledged.

3.) Anger. The repression of anger leads to changes in our physiology, which in turn lead to the development of chronic disease. However, a problem also arises if we give full vent to our anger, which can be damaging and can rebound on us in the form of such things as heart attacks and strokes. The anger dilemma is that suppressed anger is hard on our physiology over the long run, but anger expressed as rage can be immediately dangerous and even fatal. Mate suggests that when we are faced with the anger dilemma, we ask ourselves what triggered our strong emotion: "I am greatly empowered without hurting anyone if I permit myself to experience the anger and to contemplate what may have triggered it."[6] The key, therefore, is to be able to stand back from the anger and to defuse it by understanding its causes.

4.) Autonomy. In this context, autonomy means a healthy sense of self and a healthy independence. This is one of the key developmental goals for children to achieve as they grow into teenagers and then into adults. If an autonomous sense of self is established, healthy boundaries can be drawn and maintained. In 1998, The Adverse Childhood Experiences Study[7] evaluated 9,500 adults who were questioned about their childhood experiences. The researchers found that the greater the dysfunction in the family of origin, the worse the health status was in the adults, with a much greater chance of early death from heart disease, cancer, injury, and other causes. The greater the dysfunction in the family of origin, the poorer the resulting adults were at gaining autonomy and establishing healthy boundaries.

5.) Attachment. Humans cannot thrive in isolation; we all need social contact and a social network. Many studies confirm that socially isolated people have a much higher incidence of chronic illness, and that people who have a strong social network do much better, no matter what their life circumstances are. A healthy sense of attachment begins in childhood, but it is never too late to reach out to others and to become socially engaged in ways that will protect us against the ill effects of loneliness and isolation.

6.) Assertion. Relatively few people are able to assert themselves in a healthy way, but it is important to understand that we have a right to claim a place in the world and to have our basic needs met. This does not mean that we should be arrogant or bullying, which are expressions of anger and contempt rather than of autonomy. Healthy assertion means that we require our basic human dignity to be respected, and in return we are willing to respect the autonomy and dignity of others. Only then can our mutual attachment and social interdependence be properly acknowledged.

7.) Affirmation. No one is perfect, but focusing exclusively on the negative characteristics of other people soon results in cynicism and bitterness. Rather, each human person has unique gifts and creative potential, and it is energizing and revitalizing to acknowledge and affirm the positive attributes of others. Cynicism and bitterness lead eventually to isolation which, as we see, leaves us prone to illness.

These are Gabor Mate's seven steps, and I would like to add an eighth: namely, the power of forgiveness and reconciliation. When somebody wrongs us, we have a choice about what to do with the emotions that are generated. We can become angry, resentful, and hold a grudge lasting for years – or we can forgive. When we choose not to forgive, we place ourselves in a prison, and negative emotions continue to eat away at us. But if we forgive, and especially if reconciliation occurs, we are set free from the negative emotions that eventually can only do us harm. Admittedly, forgiveness and reconciliation are complex topics, dealt with by sophisticated theologians and philosophers, among others. It might therefore be pertinent for me to cite an example from my clinical practice to illustrate what I mean by forgiveness and reconciliation, but without entering into the larger debate.

Cynthia's Case

A patient of mine, Cynthia, was a single, middle-aged mother of one daughter. She was suffering from chronic fatigue, muscle pains, and anxiety. I took her through treatment with a detoxification program, which she tolerated well. She noted some improvement in her energy, and her muscle pains diminished. But her anxiety continued, and no amount of counseling or medication seemed to assist her.

As it turned out, Cynthia was the only daughter of a verbally abusive father and a mother who was also verbally abused by her husband. One summer, Cynthia traveled back to her home. As soon as she stepped through the door of her parents' house, she felt "like a little girl again," and her anxiety became suddenly worse as her father continued to be verbally abusive. But this time, Cynthia summoned up the courage to confront him about how his abusive ways had affected her over the years. When she had asserted herself and successfully declared her autonomy, she also told him that she forgave him. Something important then happened as a result of Cynthia's self-assertion and her ability to forgive. Almost immediately, she noticed a lifting of her chronic anxiety, and afterwards she continued to be relieved of this terrible burden. Over time, her relationship with her father was also restored.

Throughout this book, I have been concerned primarily with describing the effects of environmental toxins on our health. In this chapter, I have offered some brief remarks about the importance of emotional health, and in so doing I have commented on the subtle interconnections between our subjective experiences and the objective world. At this point, a vast further field of study opens before us, reaching beyond medical practice into the realms of psychology, sociology, philosophy, theology, and various humanities disciplines. No single book can address the achievements of scholars and

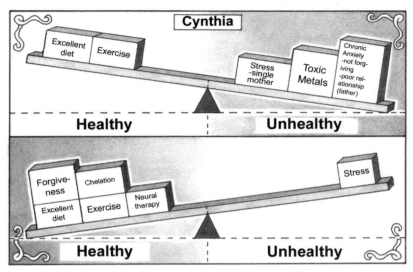

Figure 14.2 Cynthia

practitioners in these many fields. Yet one might hope to detect the signs of a consensus in the making, whereby the human person can be acknowledged anew as a complex combination of physical, emotional, and spiritual dimensions that require understanding and that must be addressed if health and well-being are truly to be promoted and enjoyed.

[1] Selye, H. The general adaptation syndrome and the diseases of adaptation. *J Clin Endocrinol.* 1946; 6:117-230.

[2] Gabor Maté, G. *When the Body Says No: The Cost of Hidden Stress.* 2004. Vintage. Canada.

[3] Selye, H. *The Stress of Life.* New York: McGrawHill, 1956. Rev. ed. 1976.

[4] Gabor Maté, G.*When the Body Says No: The Cost of Hidden Stress.* 2004. Vintage. Canada. p 263.

[5] Ibid. pp 259-281

[6] Ibid. p 273.

[7] Felitti VJ, Anda RF, et al. Relationship of childhood abuse and household dysfunction to many of the leading causes of death in adults. The Adverse Childhood Experiences (ACE) Study. Am J Prev Med. 1998 May; 14(4):245-58.

15

Summary - Putting It All Together

When new patients come to my clinic, I think in terms of the concepts presented in the preceding chapters. I can then assist these patients to discover what toxic exposures they have had, and to identify factors in their lives that may prevent them from detoxifying efficiently. I listen carefully to their life histories to get an idea of what has led to their present conditions, so that we can work to eliminate the toxic foci one at a time and gradually tilt the balance back towards health. As the preceding chapters suggest, a number of steps are usually followed for optimal detoxification to occur, and I will now summarize these steps briefly.

Minimize Exposure

The first priority is to avoid exposure to toxins as much as possible. When we are exposed, it is important to do as much as we can to ensure that the rate of biotransformation and excretion of toxins exceeds the rate of accumulation. Otherwise, toxins will gradually build and overwhelm the cellular processes, leading to disease. Recently, one of my patients, who was recovering from fibromyalgia, asked me if it would be all right for her to go back to doing her stained-glass hobby. I advised her emphatically to avoid doing so because she would be reexposed to lead fumes, and her illness would eventually recur. Often my patients ask if they can have mercury chelation therapy without removing their mercury amalgams. It is true that dental work is a major challenge and expense, but leaving the mercury amalgams in place results in ongoing and continuous exposure to mercury vapor. I usually refuse to treat patients unless they agree to get rid of the major source of their mercury – namely, their amalgams. In cases such as these, toxins simply reaccumulate faster than they are excreted, and constant vigilance is required to prevent such a thing from happening.

It is important also to minimize exposure to electromagnetic fields, especially the kind that are readily ignored in our everyday environment. As we have seen, some of these fields have sources external to the body (such as cell phones and various household appliances), and others are generated within the body (from surgical scars and the galvanic activity associated with mercury amalgams, metallic crowns, and the mixture of various metallic alloys in the mouth). It is difficult for the body to detoxify itself effectively if significant electromagnetic fields are present, and, again, vigilance is required if we are to take adequate notice of the various sources of electromagnetic contamination which we encounter from day to day.

Alkalinize the Body

The internal environment of our bodies is maintained at a pH of approximately 7.35, meaning that our internal environment is more alkaline than acidic. The large majority of chronically ill patients who come to my clinic have an acidic internal environment. This is determined by precise measurements of saliva, blood, and urine, using highly sensitive electrodes as part of the Biological Terrain Analysis,[1] although patients also can perform a simple test at home by using litmus paper to check the pH of their saliva and urine.

Maintaining a healthy alkaline state is a dynamic process that changes from moment to moment through millions of reactions that produce acidic by-products. Adequate alkaline reserves are necessary to buffer the acids produced by these reactions, and the body also requires acid-buffering minerals in adequate amounts, as well as the efficient and brisk elimination of toxic waste products. When an alkaline environment is maintained, the body's cellular processes in general function at their best, and the most effective way to keep the body in a more alkaline state is to consume a variety of alkaline rich foods.[2]

Maintain Bowel Health

I begin treatment of almost every patient by recommending interventions that will improve the integrity of the lining of the intestine. These interventions include dietary changes (such as eliminating foods that cause chronic inflammation in the lining of the intestine), treatment of overgrowths of organisms (such as parasites, fungi, and other pathogens), introduction of nutritional foods, probiotics, and possibly medical food products, as well as the use of nutritional supplements. If this important first step is neglected, patients often will feel much worse when the detoxification processes begin. This is especially true in the case of heavy metal detoxification, because once heavy metals are mobilized, they must be eliminated and excreted efficiently by way of a healthy intestine; otherwise they will redistribute to other parts of the body, causing further disruption of cellular function.

I once had an urgent telephone call from a person with multiple sclerosis, who told me that her doctor had administered DMPS intravenously and then left on holiday. Besides experiencing severe muscle cramps, she felt weak and was also having anxiety. As it turned out, her doctor was not trained in the use of DMPS, and, before being treated, the patient had been given no dietary interventions, no interventions to improve her gastrointestinal function, and no alkaline minerals to prevent muscle cramps. When I questioned her, she told me that she normally had one bowel movement per week. Promptly, I gave her advice on how to get her bowels moving, as well as advice on dietary and nutritional supplements. I also told her not to get any more DMPS until these foundational issues were addressed properly. This case demonstrates the importance of good bowel health and functioning if detoxification is to proceed effectively.

Balance Phase 1 and Phase 2 Liver Detoxification Pathways

As we have seen, it is important for the detoxification pathways in the liver to function optimally. The liver is like a large factory with several divisions that must work in a synchronized fashion if toxins are to be eliminated efficiently. For instance, if the Phase 1 pathways

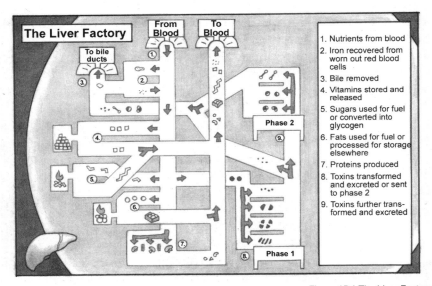

Figure 15.1 The Liver Factory

are working in overdrive and the Phase 2 pathways are working too slowly, then the toxins produced from Phase 1 cannot be shunted effectively into the Phase 2 pathways and instead are released into the body. These intermediate toxins are often more damaging to health than the original toxins, but if the gastrointestinal tract is functioning well, and if the hundreds of detoxification pathways in the liver are given the key nutrients required to build the enzymes running these pathways, then marvelous improvements in health can occur as a result of attention to these matters alone.

Phase 1 / Phase 2 – Detoxification Scenarios

1	Phase 1 (Normal)	Phase 2 (Normal) = ⇒ Toxins eliminated in bile and urine
2	Phase 1 ⬇	Phase 2 (Normal) = ⬆ Toxic Intermediates into the Body
3	Phase 1 ⬆	Phase 2 (Normal) = ⬆ Toxic Intermediates into the Body
4	Phase 1 (Normal)	Phase 2 ⬇ = ⬆ Toxic Intermediates into the Body

Figure 15.2

Eliminate Toxins

Heavy metals make up the first main group of toxins adversely affecting our health, and the top three are arsenic, lead, and mercury. POPs (Persistent Organic Pollutants) are the second main group, and the third group is biological, produced by various forms of bacteria, fungi (yeast), and parasites.

Heavy metals are best removed by a judicious use of chelating agents which bind to the metallic toxins so that they can be eliminated. The use of a far infrared sauna is especially helpful in eliminating POPs, and this relatively new technology is affordable for home use. The largest reservoir of biological toxins is the colon, which is an ecosystem unto itself and must be maintained in good working order. Another important reservoir of biological toxins is osteonecrotic lesions found in the jawbones, especially in people who have had root canal procedures or dental extractions. Proper treatment of the necrotic bone, as well as the use of red and infrared light, can be highly effective in such cases.

With the removal of harmful chemicals and heavy metals, the body becomes much less vulnerable to biological organisms of many kinds. As well, the immune system functions much better when detoxification has taken place, and this improved functioning in turn assists the body to eliminate or control the growth of harmful organisms.

These are the main concerns that I address in my day-to-day work with patients. I will close with one last case that provides an effective summation of these main concerns. Dorothy had a variety of symptoms, and her case allows us to see how wide-ranging are the hazards of our modern toxic environment, while also demonstrating that effective action can be taken against the pollutants which all too frequently are devastating to our health.

Dorothy's Case

When I first met Dorothy, she appeared tired and depressed. She told me she had spent her childhood on a farm on the prairies where she was exposed to various pesticide and herbicide sprays. As a child, she had multiple mercury amalgams placed in her teeth, but she had no root canals or crowns. She had all her wisdom teeth extracted under general anesthetic because they were impacted, and she was not aware of any complications from this procedure. She told me that when she was fourteen years old, her mother constructed a barometer, and Dorothy had played with the liquid mercury it contained.

Dorothy became a registered nurse, and she was generally healthy before going to the Philippines at age thirty to work for a period of seven years with a Christian mission. Although the water she drank in the Philippines was filtered, she suspected that it contained pathogenic organisms because she had multiple episodes of dysentery. She also had dengue fever twice, and every six months she was treated with antihelminthic (anti-worm) medications. She also took medications to prevent malaria. She was constantly bitten by mosquitoes during the rainy season, and she was aware of the great amount of air pollution caused by large numbers of vehicles using leaded gasoline. Her last year in the Philippines was spent in Manila, where she found the air pollution unbearable. Her skin deteriorated, and her hair began falling out; she also suffered from extreme fatigue and insomnia. Her work was stressful, and she began to develop problems with making decisions, partly because she had difficulty remembering and following instructions. Her hearing became hypersensitive, and she began to react to various fumes and chemicals – for instance, she developed a burning sensation in her mouth and feet. Her heart would pound when she was at rest, and she would often experience a trembling sensation within her body.

Dorothy visited a psychiatrist in Manila who placed her on an antidepressant medication, which had the effect of making her feel highly agitated. After seven years, she returned to Canada and was given a series of antidepressants (including Elavil, Prozac, Serzone, Zoloft, Paxil, and Effexor). She told me that she did not find any of these antidepressants to be helpful and that she was living a zombie-like existence. Several years went by, and she went through menopause. She was then placed on synthetic hormone replacement therapy, but her health continued to deteriorate, and out of desperation she traveled a great distance to consult with an excellent naturopathic physician. Hair analysis was performed and showed elevated levels of lead, nickel, silver, and tin. She was placed on a large number of very expensive supplements, and although she felt quite well on this program, if she discontinued the supplements, her symptom complex would return rapidly.

The naturopath discontinued Dorothy's hormone replacement therapy, and she developed severe hot flashes that interfered with her sleep. Furthermore, going off the hormone replacement therapy led to a deterioration of her cognitive function. At the time I met her, she was working as a secretary at a university, and she was finding it difficult to perform her job. She would forget to keep appointments, and she was able to perform only one task at a time. Often when she spoke, the wrong word would come out. When she wrote by hand, she often omitted letters or reversed numbers.

Dorothy then went to a neurologist who ordered an MRI scan of her brain. The MRI found two small hyperintense areas in the white matter of the frontal lobes. The conclusion was that these hyperintense areas might be related to decreased blood flow to that part of the brain, or possibly to demyelination (breakdown of the protective layer around nerves). At the same time, she was adamant that she would never go back on antidepressant medication or hormone replacement therapy.

Dorothy had a conglomeration of other symptoms, including a marked weight gain from the antidepressant medications. She would often overeat, and because of her weight gain, she snored (an overnight sleep study ruled out sleep apnea), and she often experienced restless legs during the night. She had a chronic intolerance to cold, and her body temperature was often subnormal. She had no hypoglycemia, diabetes, or cardiovascular problems. She had very few symptoms related to the gastrointestinal tract, such as burping or bloating. Since menopause, the frequency of her headaches decreased significantly, and she had no further leg cramps during the night. Over the years, she gradually had mercury amalgams replaced with composite materials. Dorothy's sister had developed Parkinson's with dementia in her late fifties, and her maternal grandmother and maternal cousin both had breast cancer.

When I examined her, Dorothy's blood pressure and pulse were normal. Her skin was very dry. She had two mercury amalgams present in her mouth. The membranes in her nasal passages were chronically swollen (implying allergies). She had tenderness above her left collarbone where the lymphatic vessels draining the head come together. She had very few tender points present throughout her musculoskeletal system (making the diagnosis of fibromyalgia less likely). The neurological exam was normal, except that she was unable to stand with one foot directly in front of the other with her eyes closed. Numerous blood tests, including serological tests for toxoplasmosis and Lyme disease, were unremarkable.

Based on her history of multiple chronic assaults on her gastrointestinal tract while in the Philippines, I gave Dorothy two medical food products, starting with RevitalX™ which she used for a period of three weeks, followed by Detoxitech™ for one week. These products are designed to rejuvenate the gastrointestinal tract and boost liver function; subsequently, Dorothy continued to use both products one or two days per week. She was also given dietary instructions that helped to alkalinize her system and she was placed on a number of supplements to prepare for a DMPS challenge test to assess the effects of her exposure to mercury and lead. The results showed excessive levels of lead (11 mcg, with normal less than 5) and mercury (51 mcg, with normal less than 4), and smaller amounts of several other metals were also elevated. (see Figure 15.3)

DETOXIFY FOR LIFE

URINE TOXIC METALS

POTENTIALLY TOXIC METALS

METALS	RESULT µg/g CREAT	REFERENCE RANGE	WITHIN REFERENCE RANGE	ELEVATED	VERY ELEVATED
Aluminum	< dl	< 35			
Antimony	0.3	< 1	▬		
Arsenic	56	< 130	▬▬		
Beryllium	< dl	< 0.5			
Bismuth	< dl	< 15			
Cadmium	0.9	< 2	▬▬		
Lead	11	< 5	▬▬▬▬▬▬		
Mercury	51	< 4	▬▬▬▬▬▬▬▬▬▬▬▬		
Nickel	6.8	< 12	▬▬		
Platinum	< dl	< 1			
Thallium	0.1	< 0.8	▬		
Thorium	< dl	< 0.3			
Tin	5.7	< 10	▬▬		
Tungsten	< dl	< 1			
Uranium	< dl	< 0.2			

CREATININE

	RESULT mg/dL	REFERENCE RANGE	2SD LOW 1SD LOW	MEAN	1SD HIGH 2SD HIGH
Creatinine	59	35- 225	▬▬▬▬▬		

SPECIMEN DATA

Comments:
Date Collected: 6/21/2004   Method: ICP-MS   Collection Period: Random
Date Received: 6/23/2004   <dl: less than detection limit   Volume:
Date Completed: 6/24/2004   Provoking Agent: DMPS   Provocation: POST

Toxic metals are reported as µg/g creatinine to account for urine dilution variations. **Reference ranges are representative of a healthy population under non-challenge or non-provoked conditions.** No safe reference levels for toxic metals have been established.   V10.00

©DOCTOR'S DATA, INC. • ADDRESS: 3755 Illinois Avenue, St. Charles, IL 60174-2420 • CLIA ID NO: 14D0646470 • MEDICARE PROVIDER NO: 148453

Figure 15.3

A Cavitat examination of Dorothy's lower jawbones was then undertaken, and this showed presumptive evidence of bilateral osteonecrosis, associated with her wisdom teeth extraction sites. Dorothy was referred to a biological dentist who carefully removed her remaining mercury amalgams. A minor surgical procedure was also undertaken to remove as much of the osteonecrotic bone as possible in the lateral lower jawbone regions. Dorothy was then fitted with an LED light unit with intense infrared and red lights, which she used for twenty minutes daily. This treatment resulted in a complete resolution of the osteonecrosis in her jawbones. Dorothy then underwent a series of monthly DMPS injections in conjunction with the use of a far infrared sauna.

On Dorothy's sixth treatment, a follow-up test was completed. (see Figure 15.4) It showed a marked improvement in metals excreted: lead was undetectable and mercury had dropped to 5.6 mcg. I then placed Dorothy on oral penicillamine, twice daily for two days per week over two months, and she continued to use the far infrared sauna twice weekly. She was also took theanine at bedtime. This is a green tea extract that has effective sedating properties without side effects. As well, because of the prolonged stress to which she had been exposed, she was placed on a homeopathic adrenal extract called Energy Flash ®, which helps to improve adrenal gland function. (see Figure 15.5)

Following the two months of penicillamine, a DMPS challenge test was completed. Dorothy's mercury level measured 6.7 mcg, and she was excreting more lead, which now measured 11 mcg. (See Figure 15.5) She told me that she felt a remarkable resurgence of energy, and that her cognitive function had improved so much that she was promoted to administrative work, which she was able to handle without any problems. She no longer experienced word-finding difficulties, her sleep was normal, and she no longer required the use of theanine. Her hot flashes were negligible, and her body temperature also improved. She stated that she was finally looking

URINE TOXIC METALS

POTENTIALLY TOXIC METALS

METALS	RESULT μg/g CREAT	REFERENCE RANGE	WITHIN REFERENCE RANGE	ELEVATED	VERY ELEVATED
Aluminum	< dl	< 35			
Antimony	< dl	< 1			
Arsenic	31	< 130	▬		
Beryllium	< dl	< 0.5			
Bismuth	< dl	< 15			
Cadmium	0.7	< 2	▬		
Lead	< dl	< 5			
Mercury	5.6	< 4	▬▬▬▬▬		
Nickel	7.3	< 12	▬▬▬		
Platinum	< dl	< 1			
Thallium	0.4	< 0.8	▬▬		
Thorium	< dl	< 0.3			
Tin	1.8	< 10	▬		
Tungsten	0.3	< 1	▬		
Uranium	< dl	< 0.2			

CREATININE

	RESULT mg/dL	REFERENCE RANGE	2SD LOW	1SD LOW	MEAN	1SD HIGH	2SD HIGH
Creatinine	46	35- 225		▬▬▬▬▬			

SPECIMEN DATA

Comments:
Date Collected:	11/19/2004	Method:	ICP-MS	Collection Period:	Random
Date Received:	11/22/2004	<dl:	less than detection limit	Volume:	
Date Completed:	11/23/2004	Provoking Agent:	DMPS	Provocation:	POST PROVOCATIVE

Toxic metals are reported as μg/g creatinine to account for urine dilution variations. **Reference ranges are representative of a healthy population under non-challenge or non-provoked conditions.** No safe reference levels for toxic metals have been established.   V10.00

©DOCTOR'S DATA, INC. · ADDRESS: 3755 Illinois Avenue, St. Charles, IL 60174-2420 · CLIA ID NO: 14D0646470 · MEDICARE PROVIDER NO: 146453

Figure 15.4

URINE TOXIC METALS

POTENTIALLY TOXIC METALS

METALS	RESULT µg/g CREAT	REFERENCE RANGE	WITHIN REFERENCE RANGE	ELEVATED	VERY ELEVATED
Aluminum	< dl	< 35			
Antimony	0.3	< 1	▬		
Arsenic	45	< 130	▬		
Beryllium	< dl	< 0.5			
Bismuth	< dl	< 15			
Cadmium	0.6	< 2	▬		
Lead	11	< 5	▬▬▬▬▬		
Mercury	6.7	< 4	▬▬▬▬		
Nickel	< dl	< 12			
Platinum	< dl	< 1			
Thallium	< dl	< 0.8			
Thorium	< dl	< 0.3			
Tin	1.8	< 10	▬		
Tungsten	< dl	< 1			
Uranium	< dl	< 0.2			

CREATININE

	RESULT mg/dL	REFERENCE RANGE	2SD LOW	1SD LOW	MEAN	1SD HIGH	2SD HIGH
Creatinine	20	35- 225	▬▬▬▬▬				

SPECIMEN DATA

Comments:

Date Collected:	2/14/2005	Method: ICP-MS	Collection Period: Random
Date Received:	2/16/2005	<dl: less than detection limit	Volume:
Date Completed:	2/18/2005	Provoking Agent: DMPS	Provocation: POST PROVOCATIVE

Toxic metals are reported as µg/g creatinine to account for urine dilution variations. Reference ranges are representative of a healthy population under non-challenge or non-provoked conditions. No safe reference levels for toxic metals have been established. V10.00

©DOCTOR'S DATA, INC. • ADDRESS: 3755 Illinois Avenue, St. Charles, IL 60174-2420 • CLIA ID NO: 14D0646470 • MEDICARE PROVIDER NO: 148453

Figure 15.5

forward to a healthy and productive life.

Case Discussion

Dorothy's exposure to toxins began at an early age while she was living on a farm, where she was exposed to various persistent organic pollutants in the form of pesticides and herbicides. She was exposed to leaded gasoline and possibly to leaded paint in the farmhouse. She began getting mercury amalgams placed in her teeth as a child, and she was further exposed when she played with liquid mercury at fourteen years old. Her impacted wisdom teeth were extracted, and although she was not aware of complications, she went on to develop hidden infections in those areas of her jawbones. Consequently, even before she went to the Philippines, the stage was set for the TILT Phenomenon to come into play when her body was subjected to additional stress. (see Figure 15.6)

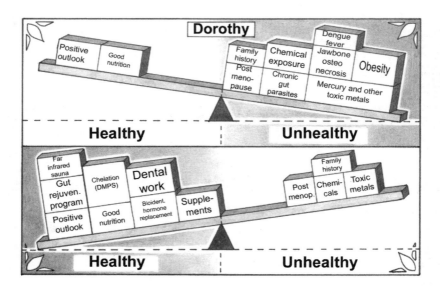

Figure 15.6 Dorothy

Conditions in the Philippines increased Dorothy's toxic burden significantly. Besides breathing heavily polluted air, she had major exposure to parasitic and worm organisms, as is evidenced by her large number of bowel infections. The fact that she had dengue fever twice also had a strongly negative impact on her system.

As Dorothy's toxic burden increased, her whole system tilted for the worse, and she did not recover until the underlying causes were found and corrected through a carefully designed and managed detoxification program. This program allowed Dorothy's whole system to rebalance, and her overall health has improved remarkably. Yet Dorothy's story of recovery is not over, and she, like the rest of us, will have to be careful to continue with a lifestyle that emphasizes ongoing detoxification.

---

[1] Vincent LC. Importance of bio-electronics for the determination of biologic terrains. Rev Fr Odontostomatol. 1965 Oct; 12(8):1235-50.

[2] Jaffe RM. Food & Chemical Effects on Acid/Alkaline Body Chemical Balance. www. elisaact.com.

Appendix A

CELL BIOLOGY

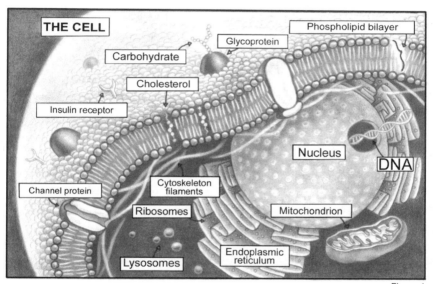

Figure 1

Throughout this book, I have focused on the detoxification therapies that affect the inner workings of our cells, which are the basic units of our bodies. I provide this appendix for readers who might be interested in having a little more information about our fascinating and beautifully complex cell biology.[1]

Each cell in our body is an organism that needs to eat, drink, breathe, and detoxify itself. Some researchers have estimated that each of us has approximately 40 trillion cells, and Figure 1 is an artist's depiction of what one of these cells looks like. Please refer to this illustration frequently as you read through this appendix.

Each cell is surrounded by an elaborate extracellular (meaning outside the cell) matrix. This matrix is highly complex and is made up of glycoproteins ("glycol" means sugar, and protein is made up of amino acids). You can think of glycoproteins as being "sugar-coated" proteins making up a matrix. The matrix in turn is bathed in extracellular fluid, and it has specialized cells that migrate and function like garbage collectors. Other migratory cells also perform maintenance tasks, constantly rebuilding and refashioning the matrix. Nerve fibers also run through the matrix, sending nerve fibrils (tiny branches of nerves) to every cell in the body, so that the matrix functions as an information superhighway that transmits information at the speed of light – much like a liquid crystal display.

It is important to realize that cells do not function in isolation but are dependent on a healthy extracellular matrix. Heavy metals can bind to the glycoproteins and nerves in the matrix, altering their function and also markedly increasing the rate of production of free radicals. As I mentioned in Chapter 2, free radicals are highly reactive molecules that are hungry for electrons and can do extensive damage to cells.

Each cell also has a membrane that is composed of phospholipids (fats) and glycoproteins, which are arranged in what is known as a phospholipid bilayer. The tiny ball-like entities on either side of the membrane are the phosphate heads connected to the lipid tails (long chains of carbon atoms). These phospholipids are placed back-to-back, much like the two pieces of bread that make up a sandwich, and the result is a "phospholipid bylayer." As with the extracellular matrix, the integrity of a cell membrane is necessary for the thousands of cellular processes within the cell to occur as they should, but again, toxins can have an adverse impact on cell membrane function. For instance, positively charged metallic toxins will readily bind to the negatively charged surface of the cell membrane, a process that causes alterations in the structure of the membrane and results in a multimillion-fold increase in production of free radicals.

Each cell membrane moves continuously like a wave, but as we age the ratios of various phospholipids change and make the cell membrane less fluid. As a result, the cell does not function as well as it should. The glycoprotein structures sticking up through the membrane are receptors (or docking stations for biochemical messages sent to the cell). The membrane, therefore, is an interface between the outside and the inside of the cell, allowing messages coming to the cell to be processed and allowing signals to be sent out, thereby commanding various further processes to occur elsewhere in the body.

An electrical gradient across the cell membrane enables these messages to be transmitted. It is vital that the transmembrane electrical gradient is maintained at 80 mV, otherwise a negative signal is sent into the cell, causing it to self-destruct. Exposure to abnormal electromagnetic fields can influence this gradient, which in turn can be restored by exposure to certain pulsating magnetic fields.

If we imagine ourselves traveling into the cell, we will now see the cytoskeleton, or scaffolding, that supports its interior. We will be surrounded by the fluid inside the cell (the cytoplasm), and we will see numerous organelles (as our bodies have organs, so our cells have organelles), all of which have specific functions.

One of these organelles is the mitochondria, which has the appearance of an earthworm. It is a power generator, and its basic function is to disassemble carbohydrates, fats, and proteins that we obtain from food, stripping the electrons from these structures and storing them for future use in molecules called ATP (Adenosine Triphosphate). Electrons are the energy currency that powers the millions of cellular reactions that occur constantly.

The number of mitochondria in each cell varies, depending on energy requirements. For example, muscle cells in the heart require a large amount of energy to be produced continuously, and the number of mitochondria increases to meet the demand. In order to get inside the mitochondria, we have to pass through another membrane, which is also composed of a phospholipid bilayer. If fatty acids are to cross this membrane, they must be carried by an amino acid called carnitine. Because such complex chemical reactions occur in the mitochondria, each step of each chemical reaction requires specialized proteins called enzymes.

An enzyme has a specific structure that must be maintained if it is to be functional. As well, each enzyme requires the presence of a cofactor bound into its structure. The cofactor is usually a mineral such as iron, copper, magnesium, zinc, selenium, or molebdynum (over eighty trace minerals are required), as well as the B vitamins. If there are deficiencies of these minerals or vitamins, the enzymes cannot function, and energy cannot be produced. Mercury, arsenic, and lead are especially harmful because they bind to the enzymes required for chemical reactions to proceed within the mitochondria. When these metallic toxins bind to an enzyme, the shape of the enzyme is altered, and it becomes dysfunctional. Energy production then decreases or completely ceases, depending on the amount of toxins present.

The nucleus is the "library" of each cell, and contains our complete genetic code. Traveling inside the nucleus, we come across helical structures – the chromosomes containing our DNA, or genetic blueprint. The DNA can be turned on or off, depending on what factors are influencing the cell membrane and what substances are allowed to enter into the cell. For instance, if the cell requires the production of certain proteins such as enzymes, the DNA unfolds, and that part of the genetic code is read, copied, and transferred outside the nucleus where protein construction occurs. The DNA is very sensitive to toxic influences and is continuously undergoing repair by specialized molecules.

The DNA is highly vulnerable, because if alterations or mutations occur in the genetic code, altered messages are sent out to the body, with potentially disastrous effects.

As we travel out from the nucleus, we come across an odd-appearing structure that looks like a long series of membranes with knob-like protrusions called ribosomes dotted on the outside. Ribosomes are tiny units that process the messages that come out of the nucleus, going on then to construct whatever proteins are required by the cell.

Next, as we move on through the cell, we come across organelles that look like oranges. These are called lysosomes, and their job is to kill invading organisms. When an organism attaches to the outer cell membrane, the phospholipid bilayer will surround the organism to form a sphere that is then taken into the cell. This sphere joins up with the lysosomal membrane (which is also a phospholipid by-layer) and the invading organism is released into the lysosome. The organism is then exposed to hydrogen peroxide, as well as to the powerful enzymes that digest it.

As we continue our journey, looking at the inside surface of the cell membrane we observe specialized channels going through it. These channels are composed of a series of specialized proteins that open and close, depending on what the cell needs at the time. Some of these channels allow nutrients to flow into the cell, and other channels allow waste products to go out. Looking further along the inner surface of the cell membrane, we observe other types of proteins that act as pumps to remove excess calcium. Other complex protein pumps will move sodium out of the cell and allow potassium into it.

A healthy cell has a range of functions that are dictated by its genetic code, as well as by outside influences such as cell-to-cell communication, availability of nutrients, and toxic substances. A healthy cell will try to maintain an internal steady state, but when the stressors are severe enough, cells will respond in a limited number of ways, as follows [2]:

Hyperplasia The number of cells can increase.

Hypertrophy The cells can become larger. Sometimes hyperplasia and hypertrophy can occur simultaneously. Often when cells are attempting to adapt to stress, they accumulate various substances such as fats, carbohydrates, and proteins, and become larger. Also, as the cells grow, they increase in number, and obesity occurs when both processes combine.

Atrophy The cells can become smaller. For example, if there is a decrease in the amount of stress to which a cell is exposed, the cell might decrease in size. We have all experienced this "use it or lose it" principle when we stop exercising and our muscles become smaller.

Altered Metabolism Cells can alter the rate at which their metabolic processes occur, either slowing down or speeding up depending on the messages coming from the outside. For example, cells in the liver can increase the speed with which drugs or toxins are handled in order to facilitate their removal from the body.

Maladaptation Cells can have a maladaptive response to stress, the ultimate example being the extreme hyperplasia or cellular replication that occurs with cancer.

In general, if cells are unable to adapt to stress, injury occurs and may or may not be reversible. If the stress is severe enough and exceeds a point of no return, then a death gene is triggered, and the cells will self-destruct. Cellular death is the ultimate result of injury to cells and can be caused by various factors such as lack of blood supply, infectious agents, various types of trauma, and toxic influences such as chemicals, drugs, and toxic metals, genetic mutations, nutritional deficiencies, and immunologic reactions.

However, our cells can also adapt successfully. For instance, exercise increases the oxidative stress to which cells are exposed, with the result that the cells respond by increasing the number of their own antioxidant enzymes, so that oxygen is handled more efficiently at the cellular level. Furthermore, when muscle cells are exercised, they proliferate and the muscle group gets larger. This also occurs in the heart if it has to pump over a long period of time against high pressure in the arteries. The heart adapts by increasing the number of heart muscle cells and by enlarging individual cells.

Cells can also adapt due to hormonal or growth factor influences. For example, under the influence of estrogen and progesterone, the lining of the uterus will grow each month during the menstrual cycle. In men, the prostate gland will become larger under the influence of androgenic hormones.

Our bodies are composed of trillions of cells that work together in a marvelous way. Each cell is intricately designed and has a complex, fascinating architecture. As we see, cells seek to maintain a steady state and, when exposed to various stressors, strive to adapt. In so doing, they seek at a microscopic level the same kind of balance that we seek as we care for the health of our bodies as a whole.

---

[1] An interactive Web site on cell biology is www.cellsalive.com.

[2] Kumar: Robbins and Cotran. Pathologic Basis of Disease, 7th ed. 2005; Saunders.

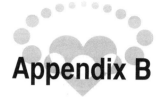

Appendix B

Comprehensive Elimination Diet [1]
© The Institute for Functional Medicine

The Comprehensive Elimination Diet is designed to clear the body of foods and chemicals to which you may be allergic or sensitive. It is designed also to improve the body's ability to handle and dispose of these harmful substances.

As the word "elimination" suggests, I will ask you not to eat certain foods and food categories. Removal of these items from your diet will allow your body's detoxification machinery, which may be overburdened or compromised, to recover and begin to function efficiently again. Your body will then be able to clear various toxins that may have accumulated as a result of such things as cigarette smoking, alcohol, drugs, unhealthy foods or beverages, and exposure to harmful environmental factors of various kinds.

I have found the Comprehensive Elimination Diet to be generally well tolerated and extremely beneficial. However, as with other diets, there is no typical or normal response. People's initial reactions are highly variable, a fact that can be attributed to physiological, mental and biochemical differences among individuals, as well as the degree of exposure to various kinds of toxins.

Most often, people who persist with the diet report increased energy, mental alertness, decrease in muscle or joint pain, and an overall improved sense of well-being. However, especially in the first week, some people report discomfort as their bodies adjust. Symptoms include changes in sleep patterns, light-headedness, headaches, joint or muscle stiffness, and changes in gastrointestinal function. Such symptoms rarely last for more than a week or so.

---

[1] Used by permission. www.functionalmedicine.org.

I realize that changing food habits can be difficult and sometimes confusing. With this in mind, I have provided sample menus, recipes, snack suggestions, and other information to make the transition a manageable process for everyone.

Introduction to the Menu Plan for the Comprehensive Elimination Diet

Eat only the foods listed under "Foods to Include," and avoid the foods shown under "Foods to Exclude" in the Comprehensive Elimination Diet Guidelines. If you have a question about a particular food, check to see if it is on the food list. You should, of course, avoid any listed foods to which you know you are intolerant or allergic.

The 7-Day Menu Plan may be used as is, or as a starting point. Notice that the plan contains suggested menus. Feel free to modify these and incorporate your favorite foods, provided they are on the accepted list.

Eliminate the excluded foods from your diet for a total of four weeks. Then reintroduce the excluded foods gradually, and observe any signs or symptoms of allergic reactions. I advise patients to reintroduce one food group at a time every four days. On the first day, the food group in question is ingested three times during the day. For example, if you were reintroducing dairy products, then you would consume dairy products three times on the first day. Over the following three days you would again exclude dairy products and observe how you are feeling. If you observe a reaction, then make a note of it in your food diary and move on to the next food group. If there is no noticeable reaction, it is unlikely that you are allergic or intolerant to that food group. If you have a reaction, remove that group of foods from your diet.

A few suggestions to assist you:

- You may use leftovers for the next day's meal or part of a meal. For instance, leftover broiled salmon and broccoli from dinner could be part of a large salad for lunch the next day.
- You might want to cook extra chicken, sweet potatoes, rice, beans, etc., and reheat these for snacking or for another meal.
- Most foods on the menu plan freeze quite well.
- Please add extra vegetables and fruits as needed. Remember that the menu is basic and requires your personal touch. Also, **this is not a calorie-restricted diet,** so use the suggested snacks as needed for hunger or cravings. Leftovers can be especially handy to eat as snacks.
- If you are a vegetarian, eliminate meats and fish and consume more beans and rice, quinoa, amaranth, teff, millet, and buckwheat.
- Breakfasts that require cooking are easiest to incorporate on your days off. Muffins can be made ahead of time, frozen, and used as needed.
- If you are consuming coffee or other caffeine-containing beverages on a regular basis, it is always wise to slowly reduce your caffeine intake rather than abruptly stop it; this will prevent caffeine-withdrawal headaches. For instance, try drinking half decaf/half regular coffee for a few days, and then slowly reduce the total amount of coffee.
- Select fresh foods whenever you can. If possible, choose organically grown fruits and vegetables to eliminate pesticide and chemical residue consumption. Wash fruits and vegetables thoroughly.
- Read oil labels – use only oils that are obtained by a "cold-pressed" method.
- If you select animal sources of protein, look for free-range or organically raised chicken, turkey, or lamb. Trim visible fat, and prepare by broiling, baking, stewing, grilling, or stir-frying. Cold-water fish (for instance, salmon, mackerel, and halibut) provide another excellent source of protein and also contain omega-3

essential fatty acids, which are important nutrients. Fish is used extensively in this diet, but if you do not tolerate fish, please consult with us – we may suggest supplemental fish oils. Avoid shellfish, as it may cause an allergic reaction.

- Remember to drink the recommended amount (at least two quarts) of plain, filtered water each day.
- Strenuous or prolonged exercise may be reduced during all or part of the program to allow your body to heal more effectively without the additional burden imposed by exercise. Adequate rest and stress reduction are also important to the success of this program.

Finally, any time you change your diet significantly, you may experience symptoms such as fatigue, headaches, or muscle aches for a few days. Your body needs time to "withdraw" from the foods you eat on a daily basis, and you may crave some of the foods that you have eliminated. **Persevere**: the uncomfortable symptoms usually do not last long, and most people feel much better after the first week or so.

Comprehensive Elimination Diet Guidelines

FOODS to INCLUDE	FOODS to EXCLUDE
Fruits: whole fruits – unsweetened, frozen or water-packed, canned fruits, diluted juices	Oranges and orange juice
Non-gluten grains and starch: brown rice, oats, millet, quinoa, amaranth, teff, tapioca, buckwheat, potato flour	Grains: wheat, corn, barley, spelt, kamut, rye, triticale
Animal protein: fresh or water-packed fish, wild game, lamb, duck, organic chicken, organic turkey	Pork, beef, veal, sausage, cold cuts, canned meats, frankfurters, shellfish
Vegetable protein: split peas, lentils, and legumes	Peanuts and peanut butter
Vegetables: all raw, steamed, sautéed, juiced, or roasted vegetables	Corn, creamed vegetables
Oils: cold-pressed olive, flax, safflower, sesame, almond, sunflower, walnut, canola, pumpkin	Butter, margarine, shortening, processed oils, salad dressings, mayonnaise, and spreads
Drinks: filtered or distilled water, decaffeinated herbal teas, seltzer or mineral water	Alcohol, coffee and other caffeinated beverages, soda pop or soft drinks
Sweeteners: brown rice syrup, agate nectar, stevia, fruit sweetener, blackstrap molasses	Refined sugar, white and brown sugars, honey, maple syrup, high fructose corn syrup, evaporated cane juice
Condiments: vinegar, all spices, including salt, pepper, basil, carob, cinnamon, cumin, dill, garlic, ginger, mustard, oregano, parsley, rosemary, tarragon, thyme, turmeric	Chocolate, ketchup, relish, chutney, soy sauce, barbecue sauce, teriyaki, and other condiments

Things to watch for:

- Cornstarch in baking powder and any processed foods
- Corn syrup in beverages and processed foods
- Vinegar in ketchup, mayonnaise and mustard (these are usually made from wheat or corn)
- Breads advertised as gluten-free which contain oats, spelt, kamut, or rye
- Amaranth and millet flake cereals; many contain oats or corn
- Many canned tunas contain textured vegetable protein which is from soy; look for low-salt versions which tend to be pure tuna, with no fillers
- Multigrain rice cakes are not just rice. Purchase plain rice cakes.

Fruits

- Apples, applesauce
- Apricots (fresh)
- Bananas
- Blackberries
- Blueberries
- Cantaloupe
- Cherries
- Coconut
- Figs (fresh)
- Grapefruit
- Huckleberries
- Kiwi
- Kumquat
- Lemons, limes
- Loganberries
- Mangos
- Melons
- Mulberries
- Nectarines
- Papayas
- Peaches
- Pears
- Prunes
- Raspberries
- Strawberries

All the above fruit can be consumed raw or juiced

Vegetables cont.

- Snow peas
- Spinach
- Squash
- Sweet potato, yams
- Swiss chard
- Tomato
- Watercress
- Zucchini

All the above vegetables can be consumed raw, juiced steamed, sautéed, or baked

Non-Gluten Grains

- Amaranth
- Millet
- Oat
- Quintoa
- Rice - brown, white, wild
- Teff
- Buckwheat

Vinegars

- Apple Cider
- Balsamic
- Red Wine
- Rice
- Tarragon
- Ume Plum

Breads & Baking

- Arrowroot
- Baking soda
- Rice bran
- Gluten-free breads
- Flours: rice, teff, quinoa, millet, tapioca, amaranth, garbanzo bean, potato, tapioca
- Rice flour pancake mix
- Mochi

Flesh Foods

- Free-range chicken,
- turkey, duck
- Fresh ocean fish, e.g., Pacific salmon, halibut, haddock, cod, sole, pollock, tuna, mahimahi
- Lamb
- Water-packed canned
- tuna (watch for added
- protein from soy)
- Wild game

Vegetables	Herbs, Spices & Extracts	Dairy Substitutes
• Artichoke • Asparagus • Avocado • Bamboo shoots • Beets, beet tops • Bok choy • Broccoflower • Broccoli • Brussels sprouts • Cabbage • Bell peppers • Carrots • Cauliflower • Celery • Chives • Cucumber • Dandelion greens • Eggplant • Endive • Kale • Kohlrabi • Leeks • Lettuce – red or green leaf, Chinese • Mushroom • Okra • Onions • Pak-choi • Parsley • Potato • Red leaf chicory • Sea vegetables –seaweed, kelp	• Basil • Black pepper • Cinnamon • Cumin • Dandelion • Dill • Dry mustard • Garlic • Ginger • Nutmeg • Oregano • Parsley • Rosemary • Salt-free herbal blends • Sea salt • Tarragon • Thyme • Turmeric • Pure vanilla extract	• Almond milk • Rice milk • Coconut milk • Oat milk *Beverages* • Herbal tea (decaffeinated) • Mineral water • Pure unsweetened fruit or • vegetable juices • Spring water *Oils* • Almond • Flaxseed • Canola • Olive • Pumpkin • Safflower • Sesame • Sunflower • Walnut

Beans	Cereals & Pasta	Sweeteners
• All beans except soy • Lentils - brown, green, red • Split peas * All the above beans can be dried or canned **Nuts & Seeds** • Almonds • Cashews • Flaxseeds • Hazelnuts (filberts) • Pecans • Pistachios • Poppy seeds • Pumpkin seeds • Sesame seeds • Sunflower seeds • Walnuts *All the above seeds can be consumed as butters and spreads (e.g., tahini)	• Cream of rice • Oats • Puffed rice • Puffed millet • Quinoa flakes • Rice pasta • 100% buckwheat noodles • Rice crackers	• Fruit sweetener (Mystic lake Dairy, or Wax Orchards, or apple juice concentrate) • Agave nectar • Molasses • Rice syrup • Stevia **Condiments** • Mustard (made with apple cider vinegar) • Nutritional yeast

Comprehensive Elimination Diet
7-Day Menu Plan

- This is a suggested day-by-day menu for one week while on the Comprehensive Elimination Diet.

- Use this menu to stimulate your own ideas, and modify it according to your own taste.

- Serving sizes in each recipe are approximate; adapt them to your own appetite.

- You may mix and match foods from different days according to your own preferences.

  - Substitutions with store-bought items are allowed as long as you avoid restricted foods. For example, many instant soups or canned soups from the health food store are okay – read labels.

- Recipes for the menu items marked with an asterisk (*) are included at the end.

DAY 1

Breakfast

Cooked whole grain cereal (oatmeal, cream of brown rice, buckwheat, teff, or quinoa flakes)

- served with rice, oat, or almond milk, cinnamon, and allowable sweetener of your choice
- garnished with chopped walnuts, almonds, hazelnuts, or toasted pumpkin seeds
- topped with fresh or frozen unsweetened fruit

Lunch

Lentil Soup* or Split Pea Soup* or black bean soup
Sesame rice crackers or rice cakes
Carrot and celery sticks
Fresh figs, plums, or cherries

Dinner

Broiled salmon
Cooked millet or baked white or sweet potato or Quinoa Salad*
Oven Roasted Veggies*
Mixed greens salad with Vinaigrette Dressing*
Crispy Rice Squares* or fresh apple

DAY 2

Breakfast

Fruit Smoothie:

- blend rice or almond milk with ½ banana and/or pineapple slice and one or two ice cubes
- add flax powder or other fiber if desired
-

Applesauce Bread* or Banana Bread*

Lunch

Asparagus Soup* (or yesterday's leftover soup)
Cabbage Salad*
Rice cakes with walnut butter
Fresh peach or pear

Dinner

Broiled lamb chop
Nutty Green Rice* or Mock Mac 'n Cheese*
Cooked veggie mix:

- steam broccoli, cauliflower, and carrots
- toss with olive oil and herbs (oregano, thyme, basil, tarragon, etc.)

Fruity Spinach Salad *

DAY 3

Breakfast

Nutri-Ola* or crispy brown rice or puffed rice or puffed millet cereal

- served with rice or almond milk, topped with sliced berries

Leftover Applesauce or Banana Bread

Lunch

Brown rice and black beans mix

- topped with flax oil
- garnished with chopped scallions and sliced avocado or Guacamole*
- Baking Powder Biscuits*
- Tropical fruit salad
- sliced mango, kiwi, and strawberries
- topped with shredded unsweetened coconut and chopped walnuts or pecans

Day 3 Cont.

DAY 3 Cont.

Dinner

Broiled or poached halibut

Baked butternut or acorn squash, sprinkled with cinnamon

Chopped zucchini, red peppers, garlic and onion sautéed in olive oil, topped with basil

Mixed green salad with Vinaigrette Dressing*

- choose greens from arugula, endive, radicchio, red leaf, romaine, butter head, Boston, cabbage, dandelion, escarole; add red cabbage, garbanzo beans, red onion, olives, carrots

Mochi Rice Squares* and fresh fruit

DAY 4

Breakfast

Sweet Potato Delight* and/or leftover Nutri-Ola* square
Cantaloupe half, filled with blueberries and sprinkled with cinnamon

Lunch

Leftover Brown Rice and Black Beans mix or
Halibut salad:

- Mixed greens of your choice
- chopped vegetables with garbanzo or kidney beans
- leftover halibut cut into chunks
- Vinaigrette Dressing

Fresh banana or leftover Crispy Rice Squares*

Dinner

Skinless chicken, oven baked or broiled, sprinkled with garlic powder and tarragon

Brown rice or wild rice or Basic Kasha* dressed with flax or sesame oil

Asparagus, cut into 1-inch pieces and stir-fried in olive oil and garlic

Gingerbread*

DAY 5

Breakfast

Mochi Rice Waffles* topped with Sautéed Apples*

Fruit Smoothie:
- blend rice or almond milk with a peach and/or raspberries and one or two ice cubes
- add flax powder or other fiber if desired

Lunch

Quinoa Salad* or Chicken salad:
- mixed greens
- leftover chicken, cut into pieces
- your choice of Guacamole* or Nutty Mayo*, Beans and Greens Soup*

Rice cakes or rice bread with Pear Honey* or unsweetened apple butter

DAY 5 Cont.

Dinner

Fresh tuna, topped with herbs (tarragon, dill, or parsley), and broiled Rice pasta with olive oil and Mock Pesto* or baked sweet potato topped with flax oil

Steamed vegetables: kale or collard greens tossed with olive oil and garlic

Mixed green salad with kidney beans and Vinaigrette Dressing

Fresh fruit salad: mango and pineapple chunks, sliced kiwi

DAY 6

Breakfast

Meal in a Muffin* Breakfast Rice Pudding*

Rice milk, oat milk, or almond milk, berries, sweetener, and pecans

Lunch

Tuna salad:

- leftover tuna mashed, and mixed with:
- hummus (from health food store)

Leftover Beans and Greens Soup*

Baking Powder Biscuits*

Fresh pear or nectarine

Dinner

Roast turkey breast or broiled turkey burger or Spiced Lentil Casserole* and/or Brown Rice and Peas*

Steamed broccoli, carrots and/or green beans topped with flax oil and herbs of choice

Baked Apple*

DAY 7

Breakfast

Toasted rice bread topped with pear butter or Rice Pancakes*
topped with pear butter or sautéed apples

Cantaloupe chunks

Lunch

Turkey salad:

- Mixed greens or mix of cannelini beans, celery, scallions, and apple chunks,
- Nutty Mayo* or hummus

Cucumber slices marinated in rice vinegar and dill

Rice crackers

Banana

Dinner

Rice Pasta Primavera* or Black Beans and Yellow Rice*
Pickled Beets*

Mixed greens salad with cherry tomatoes and Vinaigrette
Dressing

Leftover Breakfast Rice Pudding* topped with dried apples

Snack Suggestions

- Rice cakes or rice crackers spread with:
    - almond or cashew nut butter or
    - apple butter or
    - Pear Honey*

- Sesame rice crackers and hummus

- Fresh fruits (except orange)

- Fresh raw veggie wedges

- Nuts and seeds (except peanuts)

- Crispy Rice Squares* or Gingerbread*

Comprehensive Elimination Diet Recipes for 7-Day Menus

DAY 1 RECIPES

Lentil Soup – *Serves 4*

2 cloves garlic, minced
1 medium onion, chopped
2 large carrots, sliced or chopped
2 stalks celery, chopped
1½ cups red and/or green lentils, well rinsed
2 quarts water or broth
Pinch thyme or any herbs of your choice
Salt to taste

Combine first 6 ingredients and bring to boil. Add seasonings. Reduce heat to medium-low and simmer, partially covered, until lentils are soft. Green lentils need about 45 minutes to 1 hour, while red lentils only need 20-30 minutes. Puree half of the soup in the blender if you prefer a creamy soup.

Split Pea Soup – *Serves 6*

3 cups dry split peas, well rinsed
2 quarts water
1 tsp. salt
1 bay leaf
½ - 1 tsp. dry mustard
2 onions, chopped fine
4 cloves garlic, minced
3 stalks celery, chopped
2 medium carrots, sliced

Salt and pepper to taste
3 Tbsp. apple cider vinegar or rice vinegar

Combine peas, water, salt, bay leaf, and mustard in 6-quart pot. Bring to boil; reduce heat and simmer, partially covered, for about 20 minutes. Add vegetables and simmer for another 40 minutes, stirring occasionally. Add more water as needed. Add salt, pepper, and vinegar to taste.

Quinoa Salad – *Serves 8-10*

1½ cups quinoa, rinsed several times
3 cups water, or chicken broth or vegetable broth (or a combination)
1 cup fresh or frozen peas (frozen baby peas should be just defrosted)
Chopped veggies, raw or lightly steamed (broccoli, asparagus, green beans, etc.)
½ cup chopped red onion
1 pint cherry tomatoes (optional)
½ cup chopped black olives (optional)
1/3 cup olive oil
2 Tbsp. balsamic vinegar or lemon juice
1 or 2 crushed garlic cloves
2-4 Tbsp. fresh dill, chopped (or 1 Tbsp. dried dill)
2 Tbsp. chopped fresh parsley
Salt and pepper to taste

Rinse quinoa well (quinoa tastes bitter if not well rinsed). Bring 3 cups water or broth to a boil. Add rinsed quinoa and bring back to boil. Simmer uncovered for about 15 minutes, until liquid is well absorbed. Transfer to large bowl with a small amount of olive oil to prevent sticking, and allow to cool.

Meanwhile, mix together remaining oil, vinegar or lemon juice, parsley, and garlic in a small bowl. Add veggies to quinoa and toss well with dressing mixture, dill, salt and pepper. Chill before serving.

Oven Roasted Veggies – *Number of servings depend on amount of veggies used*

Use any combination of the following vegetables, unpeeled, washed, and cut into bite-sized pieces: eggplant, small red potatoes, red onion, yellow or green summer squash, mushrooms, asparagus. Toss with crushed garlic cloves and olive oil; sprinkle with rosemary, oregano, tarragon, and basil to taste. Spread in roasting pan in single layers and roast approximately 20-25 minutes at 400 degrees until veggies are tender and slightly brown, stirring occasionally. The amount of time needed depends on the size of the veggies. Salt and pepper to taste. Serve while warm, or use cold leftovers in salad.

Vinaigrette Dressing – *6 servings (approximately)*

Note: ingredient amounts in this recipe are approximate - use more or less of certain ingredients to adapt recipe to your personal taste.

¼ cup each flax and extra-virgin olive oils
3 Tbsp. balsamic vinegar (preferred because it has the richest flavor)
2-3 Tbsp. water
1 tsp. dry mustard
1-3 cloves fresh garlic (whole pieces for flavor or crushed for stronger taste)
Salt and pepper to taste
Oregano, basil, parsley, tarragon, or any herbs of your

choice, fresh or dried

Place vinegar, water and mustard in a tightly capped jar, and shake well to thoroughly dissolve mustard. Add oil and remaining ingredients and shake well again. Refrigerate, and shake well before using. Dressing will harden when cold; allow 5-10 minutes to reliqueify.

Crispy Rice Squares – *Makes 2 dozen*

1 tsp. cold-pressed canola oil
½ cup brown rice syrup
2 Tbsp. sesame tahini or almond butter
3 tsp. vanilla extract
2 cups crispy brown rice cereal
2 cups puffed rice
2 cups puffed millet or Perky's Nutty Rice
½ cup pumpkin or sunflower seeds
½ cup currants, chopped dried apple, or dates

Heat oil in a large pot; add rice syrup and tahini or almond butter. Stir until bubbly. Remove from heat and stir in vanilla. Add remaining ingredients and mix well with a wooden spoon. Press into an ungreased 13 x 9-inch pan and press mixture flat. Let mixture set at room temperature or refrigerate. Cut into squares. Store in an airtight container.

DAY 2 RECIPES

Applesauce Bread – Yields 14 slices

1 cup teff flour
1 cup oat or rice flour
1 tsp. baking soda
½ tsp. cinnamon
¼ tsp. salt
¼ tsp. nutmeg
1 cup unsweetened applesauce
1 Tbsp. safflower or sesame oil
½ cup brown rice syrup or fruit juice concentrate
Egg Replacer* to equal 1 egg *(refer to recipe on page 25)*
3-4 Tbsp. apple butter
1 tsp. pure vanilla extract

Combine the dry ingredients in a large bowl. Combine the wet ingredients in a small bowl and mix into the dry ingredients. Pour into oiled 9-inch square pan. Bake at 350 degrees for 30 minutes.

Banana Bread – *Yields 14 slices*

¼ cup walnuts, ground finely in blender
1¾ cups brown rice flour
½ cup arrowroot
2 tsp. baking soda
¼ tsp. salt
½ cup chopped walnuts
1½ cups ripe mashed banana
¼ cup safflower or sesame oil
6 Tbsp. apple juice concentrate

Egg Replacer* to equal 2 eggs *(refer to recipe on page 25)*
1 tsp vanilla extract

Preheat oven to 350 degrees. Mix finely ground walnuts with flour, arrowroot, baking soda, and salt in a large bowl. Stir in the chopped walnuts. In a separate bowl, mix together the banana, oil, apple juice, egg replacer, lemon and vanilla. Add to the flour mixture and stir until just moistened. Do not over mix. Pour into a greased 9 x 5-inch loaf pan and bake for 55-60 minutes, or until cake tester inserted in middle comes out clean. Cool in pan for 10 minutes, then remove from pan and cool on wire rack.

Asparagus Soup – *Serves 4*
Used with permission from The Allergy Self-Help Cookbook, *Marjorie Hurt Jones, R.N. Rodale Press, Emmaus, Pa.*

1 lb. asparagus, trimmed
2 medium leeks or 4 large shallots
1 Tbsp. oil
2-3 cloves garlic, minced
2 cups water or chicken stock
1 tsp. dried dill weed
Pinch nutmeg

Slice off the tips of the asparagus and reserve them. Cut the remaining stalks into 1-inch pieces. Slice the leeks in half lengthwise and wash under cold water to remove any sand. Slice into ¼-inch pieces. Sauté the leeks or shallots in the oil over medium heat until soft. Add the garlic and sliced asparagus stalks. Cook, stirring, another minute or two. Add the water or stock and dill. Simmer 10-12 minutes.
Remove from heat; allow to cool 5-10 minutes. Puree half the volume at a time. Return to pan, add the reserved asparagus

tips and simmer 3-5 minutes or until tips are just barely tender. Add nutmeg. If soup is too thick, thin with additional water or stock.

Cabbage Salad – *Serves 4-6*

1 small to medium head red cabbage, thinly sliced (or use half red and half green cabbage)
8 sliced radishes or 1 grated carrot
3 green apples, diced
1 stalk celery, chopped
½ cup chopped walnuts or pecans
Dash garlic powder
2 Tbsp. olive oil
2 tsp. vinegar
1 tsp. lemon juice

Mix all ingredients in a bowl and allow to sit for an hour, stirring once or twice. Serve cold or at room temperature.

Nutty Green Rice – *Serves 4*

1 cup brown basmati rice
2 cups water
¼ to ½ tsp salt
½ cup almonds
1 bunch parsley
1 clove garlic
1½ Tbsp. lemon juice
1½ Tbsp. olive oil
½ cucumber, diced
Pepper to taste

Bring water to a boil, add rice and salt, stir and simmer, covered, for 45 minutes. Remove from heat and let sit for another 10 minutes; then remove cover and allow to cool. While rice is cooking, blend almonds, parsley, garlic, and oil in food processor. When rice is cool, stir with nut mixture, and add pepper to taste. Garnish with cucumber if desired.

Mock Mac 'n Cheese – Servings depend on amounts of ingredients used

Cook desired amount of brown rice pasta according to package instructions.
Toss cooked pasta with olive oil and sprinkle with several tablespoons of nutritional yeast.
The yeast gives the pasta a cheese-like taste.

Fruity Spinach Salad – *Serves 6-8*

1 lb. fresh spinach, washed, dried, and torn into pieces
1 pint fresh organic strawberries or raspberries, washed
½ cup chopped walnuts or sliced almonds

Dressing:
2 Tbsp. sesame seeds
1 Tbsp. poppy seeds
2 scallions, chopped
¼ cup flaxseed oil
¼ cup safflower oil
¼ cup balsamic vinegar

Cut berries in half and arrange over spinach in serving bowl. Combine dressing ingredients in blender or food processor and process until smooth. Just before serving, pour over salad and toss. Garnish with nuts.

DAY 3 RECIPES

Nutri-Ola (Basic Recipe) – *Serves 10*
Adapted with permission from Sally Rockwell's Allergy Recipes, *Nutrition Survival Press, Seattle, Washington*

2 cups arrowroot or millet flour or finely ground filberts, pecans, almonds, walnuts or sesame seeds
1 cup filberts or walnuts, coarsely ground
1 cup whole sesame seeds or sunflower seeds (or a combination)
1 cup (combined) finely chopped dried apples, papaya, apricots, currants
½ cup fruit puree or frozen fruit concentrate
½ cup sesame, or walnut or sunflower oil
2 tsp. pure vanilla or almond extract

Preheat oven to 275 degrees. Use blender or food processor to grind nuts, grains or seeds to desired consistency. Mix the nuts, seeds and/or grains in a large bowl. Mix with fruit and sweetener, oil and vanilla. Pour over the dry mixture and stir lightly. Spread mixture into a lightly oiled 15 x 10 x 1-inch baking pan. Bake for 1 hour, stirring every 15 minutes. Cool. Break into small pieces for cereal or large chunks for snacks.

Breakfast Bars
Add Egg Replacer* to equal 2 eggs *(refer to recipe on page 25)* to Nutri-Ola (Basic Recipe above):
Slowly add additional water to make a stiff batter. Follow above directions, but spread into an 8 or 9-inch square pan (ungreased) and bake at 350 degrees about 30 minutes. Cut

into squares when done.

Guacamole – *Makes 1½-2 cups*
Used with permission from The Allergy Self-Help Cookbook,
Marjorie Hurt Jones, R.N. Rodale Press, Emmaus, Pa.

2-3 ripe avocados
¼ cup chopped onions
¼ tsp. vitamin C crystals
1 Tbsp. water
1 small clove garlic, chopped

Cut the avocados in half, remove the pits, then scoop the
flesh into a blender or food processor. Add the onions, vitamin
C crystals, water, and garlic. Process until smooth. Transfer to
a small bowl. Cover and chill. Use within 2-3 days. To prevent
darkening, coat top with a thin layer of oil. For a chunky
version, mash the avocado with a fork and finely chop onions
and garlic.

Baking Powder Biscuits – *Makes one dozen*

1½ cups brown rice flour
½ cup tapioca flour
4 tsp. baking powder
1/8 tsp. salt
3 Tbsp. safflower or sesame oil
1 cup applesauce, unsweetened

Preheat oven to 425 degrees. In a medium-large mixing bowl,
stir together dry ingredients. Sprinkle oil on top and mix well
with a pastry blender or fork, until consistency is crumbly.
Mix in applesauce and stir until blended. Spoon heaping
tablespoonfuls onto ungreased cookie sheet. With spoon,

lightly shape into biscuit.

Bake 15-18 minutes until slightly browned. Serve warm for best flavor, but may be lightly reheated in a microwave.

DAY 4 RECIPES

Basic Kasha – *Serves 4-5*

1 cup buckwheat groats
2 cups water, chicken or vegetable broth
Roast the dry buckwheat groats over medium heat in a dry skillet, stirring until the grains begin to smell toasty, about 2 minutes. Add the water or broth, cover and simmer for 20-30 minutes, until kasha is tender but not mushy. Pour off any excess liquid.
Optional: add onion, garlic, and herbs to the dish.

Sweet Potato Delight – *Serves 1-2*
Adapted and used with permission from The Allergy Self-Help Cookbook, *Marjorie Hurt Jones, R.N. Rodale Press, Emmaus, Pa.*

2-4 Tbsp. chopped nuts
1 ripe banana
1 medium sweet potato, cooked
1 tsp. oil
1 Tbsp. fruit sweetener, molasses, or brown rice syrup (optional)
In a large frying pan, dry roast the nuts over medium heat for a few minutes. Shake the pan often. Cut the banana in half lengthwise. Cut the cooked sweet potato into ½-inch pieces. Add the oil to the pan. Push the nuts to the outer edges. Place the banana pieces, flat sides down, in the pan. Add the sweet

potatoes. Cover and cook for 2 minutes. Uncover, and cook for 5 minutes, until everything is heated through and browned on one side. Add the sweetener before serving.

Gingerbread – *9 squares*
Adapted with permission from Gluten-Free, Sugar-Free Cooking, *Susan O'Brien, copyright © 2006, Da Capo Press, New York.*

½ cup pecans or walnuts, finely chopped
½ cup agave nectar (preferred) or fruit sweetener
¼ cup canola oil
Egg Replacer to equal 2 eggs* *(refer to recipe on page 25)*
1 tsp vanilla
1½ cups brown rice flour
½ tsp salt
1 tsp baking powder
1 tsp baking soda
2 tsp ginger
1½ tsp cinnamon
¼ tsp nutmeg
1/8 tsp cloves
½ tsp orange rind
1 cup unsweetened applesauce

In a large mixing bowl, combine the agave nectar and oil. Beat on high speed until thoroughly blended. Add in the eggs, one at a time. Be sure to beat well between eggs. Add in the orange rind and vanilla and continue to blend together. Set aside.

Meanwhile, preheat the oven to 350 degrees and spray a 9 x 9-inch square pan with a nonstick spray. Sift together the dry ingredients and add the nuts. Add some of the dry ingredients to the wet ingredients, a little at a time, blending well. Add in ¼ cup of the applesauce, blend, then add in more flour. Continue this process until you have added all of the ingredients.

Pour the batter into the prepared pan and bake for 20-25 minutes, or until the gingerbread is done. Check for doneness by inserting a toothpick, or touching lightly on the center. Freezes well.

DAY 5 RECIPES

Mochi Rice Waffles – *Serves 4*

Purchase 1 package of cinnamon-apple Mochi and defrost.
Cut into quarters. Slice each quarter across to form 2 thinner squares.
Place one square into preheated waffle iron and cook until done.
Top with your choice of fruit or Sautéed Apples *(below)*.

Sautéed Apples – *Serves 2*

2 apples, washed
½ Tbsp. safflower oil or canola oil
2 tsp. cinnamon
2-3 Tbsp. apple juice

Thinly slice apples and sauté in oil until softened. Add cinnamon and apple juice and simmer, stirring, uncovered for a few more minutes.

Beans and Greens Soup – *Serves 4-5*

2 cups cooked white beans
2 Tbsp. olive oil
2 medium cloves garlic, crushed
1 large onion, chopped
1 bay leaf
1 stalk celery, diced
2 medium carrots, diced
1 tsp. salt
Fresh black pepper
6 cups water, vegetable, or chicken broth
½ lb fresh chopped escarole, spinach, chard, or collards (or a combination)

In a 4-6 quart soup pot, sauté the onions and garlic in olive oil over low heat. When onions are soft, add bay leaf, celery, carrot, salt, and pepper. Stir, and sauté another 5 minutes. Add broth or water and cover. Simmer about 20 minutes. Add cooked beans and your choice of greens. Cover and continue to simmer, over very low heat, another 15-20 minutes. Serve immediately or refrigerate and reheat.

Pear Honey – Makes 3 pints

Used with permission from The Allergy Self-Help Cookbook, *Marjorie Hurt Jones, R.N. Rodale Press, Emmaus, Pa.*

15 very ripe pears
½ cup water
½ cup brown rice syrup or fruit juice sweetener

Peel, quarter, and core the 15 pears. Place 12 of the pears in a stainless steel or enamel Dutch oven or 3 quart saucepan. Coarsely chop the remaining 3 pears. Place them and the water in a blender. Process until pureed. Pour into the pan with the pear quarters.

Bring to a boil, then reduce the heat to a simmer. Stir in the sweetener. Cook until pears are tender, about 30 minutes. Puree the cooked fruit in batches using a blender or food processor. The puree should be about the consistency of honey. If too thin, return it to the pan and boil it down a bit. If too thick, dilute with a little juice. Pour into jars, and store in the refrigerator for up to 1 month.

Mock Pesto – Makes 1 cup

Used with permission from The Allergy Self-Help Cookbook, *Marjorie Hurt Jones, R.N. Rodale Press, Emmaus, Pa.*

1 large ripe avocado
1 cup basil leaves
¼ tsp. lemon juice
1 garlic clove, minced or 1/8 tsp. garlic powder
¼ cup pine nuts
½ tsp. olive or flax oil

Cut the avocado in half and remove the pit. Scoop out the flesh and place it in a bowl of a food processor. Add the basil, vitamin C crystals, garlic, and pine nuts. Process for about 2 minutes – scrape the bowl as necessary. Transfer it to a small bowl, and coat the surface with oil to prevent browning. Chill.

DAY 6 RECIPES

Breakfast Rice Pudding – *Serves 4_*

1 cup uncooked short grain brown rice
1¼ cups coconut milk
1¼ cups water
½ tsp. salt
1 Tbsp. brown rice syrup
1 tsp. cinnamon
Chopped almonds or sunflower seeds <u>or</u> other nuts of choice (optional)

Combine water and coconut milk in heavy pot; bring to boil, adding rice and salt. Simmer, covered (do NOT stir) for about 45 minutes or more, until liquid is mostly absorbed and rice is soft. Remove from heat and allow to cool for 15 minutes. Stir in brown rice syrup and cinnamon, and top with nuts or seeds as desired.

Meal in a Muffin – *Makes one dozen*
Adapted with permission from Wheat-Free Sugar-Free Gourmet Cooking *Sue O'Brien, Gig Harbor, WA, 2001*

1 medium carrot, grated
1 large apple, grated
¼ cup canola oil
¼ cup unsweetened applesauce
Egg Replacement to equal 2 eggs *(refer to recipe on page 25)*
1/3 cup Mystic Lake Dairy sweetener
2 tsp. vanilla
¼ cup garbanzo bean flour
½ cup brown rice flour

¼ tsp. cinnamon
½ tsp. baking powder
¼ tsp. ginger
1/8 tsp. nutmeg
¼ cup shredded unsweetened coconut
½ cup dates

Preheat oven to 375 degrees. Mix together all wet ingredients and set aside. In a separate bowl, mix dry ingredients, then mix both together. Lightly coat muffin tins with oil spray. Fill 3/4 full and bake 15-20 minutes, or until toothpick comes out clean. Allow to cool on a rack.

Spiced Lentil Casserole – *Serves 4*

1 ½ cups lentils, rinsed well
2 Tbsp. sesame oil
3 cloves garlic, crushed
1 stalk celery, chopped
1 large onion, chopped
½ tsp. salt
1 cup shredded, unsweetened coconut
½ tsp. cinnamon
½ tsp. powdered ginger
½ tsp. turmeric
2 large green apples, washed and diced

Simmer lentils, covered, in 2½ cups water for 30-40 minutes, until tender. While they are cooking, in a wok or heavy skillet, sauté remaining ingredients, except apples, in oil until tender. Add water as necessary. Add apples, and cook 10 more minutes covered. Combine with cooked lentils in a casserole dish.

Brown Rice and Peas – *Serves 4*

Add 1 cup of green peas (either fresh and lightly steamed or frozen and just defrosted baby peas) to 2 cups of cooked brown rice. Top with your favorite herbs and add flax oil to taste.

Baked Apple – *Serves 6*

1/3 cup golden raisins
2 Tbsp. apple juice
6 cooking apples, cored
1½ cups water
¼ cup frozen unsweetened apple juice concentrate
2 tsp. pure vanilla extract
1 tsp. cinnamon
1 tsp. arrowroot

Remove peel from top third of each apple and arrange in a small baking dish. In a medium saucepan, combine other ingredients and bring to a boil, stirring frequently. Reduce heat and simmer 2-3 minutes, until slightly thickened. Distribute raisins, filling centers of each apple. Pour sauce over apples and bake, uncovered, at 350 degrees for 1 to 1½ hours. Baste occasionally, and remove from oven when apples are pierced easily with a fork. Spoon juice over apples and serve warm.

DAY 7 RECIPES

Rice Pancakes – *Makes approximately 14 (4-inch) pancakes*

1 1/3 cups rice flour
½ cup oat or millet flour
2 tsp. baking powder
½ tsp. baking soda
¼ tsp. salt
1 Tbsp. apple butter
1 Tbsp. safflower or sesame oil
Egg Replacer to equal 2 eggs *(Refer to recipe on page 25)*
1½ cups almond, oat, or rice milk
1½ Tbsp. white vinegar

Mix the almond or rice milk with the vinegar and allow them to stand for 5 minutes, until curdles form. Mix dry ingredients together and set aside. In large mixing bowl, beat apple butter, oil, egg, and milk. Add dry mixture and stir gently. Be careful not to overmix. Serve with Sautéed Apples *(refer to recipe on page 21)*.

Nutty Mayo – *Makes 1¼ cups (keeps well for 3 weeks)*
Adapted and used with permission from The Allergy Self-Help Cookbook, *Marjorie Hurt Jones, R.N. Rodale Press, Emmaus, Pa.*

½ cup cashews or other nuts
¾ cup water
3 Tbsp. vinegar
2 Tbsp. oil
1 Tbsp. arrowroot

1 Tbsp. brown rice syrup
1 Tbsp. minced parsley
1 Tbsp. snipped chives
1½ tsp. dry mustard

Grind the nuts to a fine powder in a blender. Add the water, blend 1 minute to make sure the nuts are fully ground. Add the vinegar, oil, arrowroot, sweetener, and seasonings. Blend until very smooth. Pour into a saucepan and cook a few minutes, until thick. Allow to cool; transfer to a glass jar. Store in the refrigerator.

Rice Pasta Primavera – *Serves 4*

2 cups uncooked rice pasta (noodles, spaghetti, elbows)
1 large whole chicken breast, cut into thin strips (optional)
Broccoli florets, chopped carrot, and/or other favorite veggies, lightly steamed
3-4 scallions, chopped
2 cloves garlic, minced
1 Tbsp. olive oil (more if needed)
¼ cup fresh basil, finely chopped
¼ - ½ cup coconut milk

Cook rice pasta according to package directions. While pasta is cooking, heat oil in wok or heavy frying pan, and stir-fry chicken strips or tofu chunks, garlic, scallions, and basil for about 5 minutes. Add remaining vegetables and coconut milk, and continue to cook until veggies are soft and glistening. Add more coconut milk as needed. Remove from heat, and spoon over drained rice pasta. Garnish with black olives and extra olive oil, if desired.

Black Beans and Yellow Rice – *Serves 4*
Black Beans
   1 cup dry black beans, soaked overnight and drained
   4 cups water
   1 small onion, chopped
   1 small carrot, chopped
   2 cloves garlic, minced
   1 bay leaf
   1 tsp. cumin

In a 3-quart saucepan, combine beans, water, onion, carrot, green pepper, jalapeno pepper, garlic, bay leaf, cumin, and pepper flakes. Bring to a boil over medium heat and simmer, uncovered, about 2½ hours, or until beans are tender and almost all liquid is absorbed. Discard bay leaf. (May be made up to 2 days ahead; reheat before serving.)

Yellow Rice
   2 cups chicken stock
   1 small onion, finely chopped
   2 tsp. olive oil
   1 clove garlic, minced
   ½ tsp. turmeric
   1 cup uncooked long-grain brown rice

In a 2-quart saucepan over low heat, sauté onions in oil until tender, about 5 minutes. Add the garlic and sauté 1 minute. Stir in turmeric, then rice. Add stock. Bring to a boil, cover and simmer 45 minutes over low heat, or until rice is tender and all liquid is absorbed. Do not stir. Spoon beans over rice.

Pickled Beets – *Serves 4-6*
Adapted with permission from The Allergy Self-Help Cookbook,
Marjorie Hurt Jones, R.N. Rodale Press, Emmaus, Pa.

4 beets, cooked and skinned
¼ cup water
1 Tbsp. brown rice syrup or fruit sweetener
¼ cup rice vinegar
¼ tsp. ground cinnamon
Pinch each of cloves and allspice

Combine the water, sweetener, vinegar, cinnamon, cloves and allspice in a medium saucepan. Simmer for 2 minutes. Stir in the beets, and heat through. Serve hot or warm.

Miscellaneous Recipes

Egg Replacer – *equals one egg*

1/3 cup water
1 Tbsp. whole or ground flaxseed

Place the water and flaxseed together and allow to gel for about 5 minutes. This mixture will bind patties, meat loaves, cookies, and cakes as well as eggs do, but it will not leaven like eggs for souffles or sponge cakes. Increase amounts accordingly for additional egg replacement.

Corn-Free Baking Powder

2 tsp. cream of tartar
2 tsp. arrowroot
1 tsp. baking soda

Sift together to mix well. Store in an airtight container. Make small batches.

Baking Tips

- We include ground nuts in addition to chopped nuts in the muffin recipes, because the nuts help retain moisture and allow for a small amount of leavening.

- To grind soft nuts such as walnuts or pecans, use 1-2 Tbsp. of the starch called for in the recipe and add to the grinding mixture to prevent clumping.

  The grinding may be done with a nut chopper, a small (very clean) coffee grinder, or by pulsing on a food processor. Particles should be fine enough to pass through a strainer. Grind only what you will need. If you are allergic to nuts, replace the amount of nut flour with an equal amount of another flour or starch called for in the recipe.